Let Me Die Laughing!

Waking From The Nightmare Of A Brain Explosion

Megan Timothy

Crone House Publishing

Copyright © 2006 Megan Timothy

Crone House Publishing
PO Box 1856
Idyllwild, CA 92549-1856
951.659.1938
www.cronehousepublishing.com

ISBN: 1-932905-06-5

Printed in the United States of America
First Edition
  2 3 4 5 6 7 8 9 10

Book and cover designed by Rachel McMaster
Cover art by Jennifer J. Jones

Unless otherwise noted, all photographs and article reprints are courtesy of the author.

FOREWORD
by the Publisher

SERENDIPITY

*The faculty of finding valuable
or agreeable things not sought for.*

*You might argue that it's possible to lead an entirely
serendipitous life – simply don't expect or seek anything
in particular and most of what happens then appears to
be the result of serendipity. On the other hand, having
almost no expectations might also lead to a stagnant life
– one with little depth or meaning. The trick, I believe, is
to find the balance between being without expectations of
any sort and having such strong, overwhelming desires
that life constantly disappoints you.*

The author of this book, Megan Timothy, has
had a life that has been anything but boring. She
was born in Rhodesia, in Southern Africa, and came
to the U.S. when she was 20. Megan's done things
like owning her own turn-of-the-century B & B in
N. Hollywood, for which she went to culinary school
and became a chef specializing in fantasy wedding
cakes.She rafted down the Mississippi and traveled
along much of the Amazon. She biked 10,000 miles
around Europe (<u>when she was 56!</u>) and worked for a
number of years as an actress and screenwriter in
Hollywood. Not boring!

Megan cared for her very ill mother until Mum's
death, which left Megan in financial ruin. A close
friend offered her a cottage on a small ranch in return
for Megan's help with the animals and gardening.

They both saw this as an opportunity for Megan to fall back and regroup, but nature had a different path laid out for Megan. The very day she moved to the ranch, Megan suffered an aneurism in her brain. This left her unable to speak or to read or to write. She was dropped into a prison of non-communication by a cruel joke of nature.

Her story of waking up in the hospital unable to convey to those around her what she was thinking is frightening. She further tells of spending a couple of weeks in "rehab", actually a state mental hospital - terrifying! As you read this book, keep in mind that just a year ago the author could barely put a sentence together on paper.

With a deep sense of awe, I read the pages of Megan's manuscript. In gratitude for the gift I've been given, I offered her a contract to publish this book. With peels of laughter she and I have shared our life stories over cups of hot tea and contraband chocolate candy during the months we've worked together to bring her story to you.

Megan and I both believe in miracles. We know that what our Minds and our Souls are determined to achieve will come to pass. We just have to stand still long enough for the miracles to occur and they will. Much of the time we have to get out of the way of our own best intentions and let the Universe work on our behalf.

Early in our working relationship, I sent Megan a small piece I'd recently written to help keep her spirits up as she struggled to complete the second half of the manuscript. She and I have both adopted this as our "Writer's Creed".

The Power
Of The Written Word –
A Writer's Creed

Writing empowers me to be better today
    than I was yesterday.
It can also create in me an obsessive need
    for perfection.
When I write something
    that totally connects with my Soul,
    it's both the most healing and, at times,
    the most terrifying experience I know.
I write because I live.
I live because I write.
This is not a paradox.
It's the rules of engagement for my life.

N. Layton

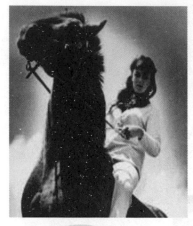

An avid horsewoman from childhood, Megan used that skill to help land parts in Hollywood movies.

Megan poses in front of the Tower of Piza on her 10,000 mile solo bike ride around Europe, the Middle East, and N. Africa

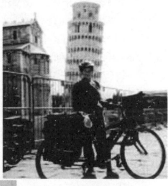

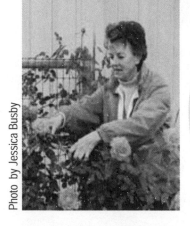

Photo by Jessica Busby

Megan loves gardening and has grown many flowering and edible plants around her cottage at the Hemet ranch owned by her friend, Jaki.

INTRODUCTION

For me, to follow just one road through life would be to suffocate. My lust for living demands a thousand paths leading to unexpected experiences. One great meal after another. Each tantalizingly different, for who wants to eat the same thing everyday, even if it's cake.

I'm accused of being a rolling stone since I fail to gather moss. If moss be money and material possessions, it's true. My stone rolls far and wide, and rather than being blanketed with moss, it's polished as smooth and shiny as a gemstone. It glows with experience, sparkles with adventure, dazzles with challenges to both mind and body, gleams with eager anticipation of the next quest. How much richer do I deserve to be?

My current journey is not one of my choosing but one that has been given to me. Two years ago I suffered an AVM (arterial venous malformation), a silent, hidden, congenital defect that triggered a bleed in my brain similar to a stroke. It robbed me of my speaking, reading, and writing abilities, and without communicative skills you are imprisoned within the solitary confinement of your mind.

My journey home has been, and continues to be, long, difficult and sometimes tainted with bitter fruit. But there are also sweet cherries to be found along the way.

The trick is to remember to spit out the pits.

To
Jaki and Sue,
who so generously gave me
two years of their lives
that enabled me
to regain mine!

2nd September 2003

I wake up sitting on the edge of my bed
How did I get here
Why does my head ache
A row of peculiar blue yellow and red
    labels stick to my left side
Who put them there
Why can't I peel them off or at least read
    the writing
My head hurts
Is it a hangover
Can't be, I don't drink
I stagger to the kitchen for an ice pack to
    relieve my headache and ease the
    unrelenting desert heat
The colored labels remain stuck to my
    head
I'm confused
The full moon offers no answers
I return to bed to sleep it off
Night disappears
Daylight comes and goes

Darkness brings anxious friends who fail to understand anything I say even though I repeat myself again and again

What's wrong with them

While my head is still groggy it doesn't hurt anymore

My friend, Jaki, calls 911 for an ambulance

"What for?" I argue

She still acts as if she doesn't understand me

Why is she being so difficult

If I'm going to the hospital then I must put on my best underwear

I insist

And shouldn't I at least shave my legs

Jaki hasn't a clue what I'm saying and demands I sit still

I only manage the underwear before the paramedics arrive

The blinding hospital lights sear my
   eyes
It doesn't matter
My eyes, and in fact my entire body,
   are no longer of significance to me
Only my thoughts matter
Only they are important
I flutter like a caged bird desperate to
   escape this heavy obsolete body -
   desperate for the freedom to fly to
   some far-off place
Jaki runs alongside my gurney barely
   keeping up
Death is in a hurry
"Jaki," I cry out in surprise "I'm dying!"
I try to tell her she's welcome to all my
   earthly stuff
But again she doesn't understand
And she's drifting away
So far away

A white door slams in her face
She's gone

I'm drifting too
Is this all there is to death
An odd floating sensation
I'm disappointed and annoyed having
    expected drama excitement and an
    impressive production
Who invited Death anyway
Not me
How dare he barge in
What about my book half- written
All the places yet to explore

And most of all friends I haven't taken the
    time to say I love

Too late now

Where Am I?

Where am I?

Am I dead?

I see Jaki and my friend Sue floating
    around

Maybe they're really angels only I never
    knew it

A young woman holding a handful of
    fruit asks me to name a banana

She won't give it to me because I call it
    "chicken"

Why on earth do I call it "chicken"?

Too tired to find the answer I fall asleep

Where am I?

It appears Death has a sense of humor

He's dressed me up like a Christmas tree

I'm festooned with yards of streamers
    and blinking lights

Jaki and Sue float around with the
    woman and her bananas

And there's a man who asks me to recite
      the alphabet and tell him the day and
      date
I think he really wants me to sing a
      Christmas carol
I try but the only words that come out are
      "chicken" followed by a slew of
      obscenities
I weep and swear and drift back to sleep

Where am I?

I hear Jaki's voice
She says something about me moving
Moving where?
Dead people don't move
I'm too tired and confused to understand
All I want to do is sleep

I'm startled awake
Two strange men drag me onto a gurney
I yell

They don't appreciate being told to do
    something impossible and indecent
    to a chicken
I try to sit up but find I'm restrained
It's impossible to move
Panic
I can't seem to breathe
Sweat streams down my neck
Survival kicks in
Missing pieces of my mind click into
    place
"Untie me!" I demand
So, there is more to my life than
    "chicken"!
 Maybe
"Policy or not, I don't want to be bound," I
    mean to say
But instead of words the obscene
    "chicken" returns and the men ignore
    me
I try to curb my panic and confusion

The softly lit hallways of a hospital are
    empty

The elevator's glaring light is spearing
    my head
I clamp my eyes shut but the light
    pierces through
My bound hands are unable to protect
    my eyes
To struggle is useless
To try to speak is useless
I choke back my screams and swallow
    my anger

A single ambulance waits in the hot,
    dark night
"Where are you taking me?" I cry out in
    fear
But my words come out all wrong and
    the men continue to ignore me

The ambulance door slams shut melting me
    away to nothing

Zero

Along with me, everything and everyone I ever
    knew disappears

Driving To Nowhere

"Cadunck", "cadunck", "cadunck"
The tires sing as they whip over the
    freeway cats-eyes
"Cadunck", "cadunck", "cadunck"
Tall amber street lights and a brazen
    army of halogen headlights
    overwhelm the night sky
"Cadunck", "cadunck", "cadunck"!
It's a long, long way to nowhere
"Cadunck", "cadunck", "cadunck"!
I'm too tired to panic
"Cadunck", "cadunck", "cadunck"!
Too tired to fight
"Cadunck", "cadunck", "cadunck"!
Too tired to think
"Cadunck", "cadunck", "cadunck"!

The ambulance slows
The noise dies down
The bright lights fade
The man sitting beside me places a note
    in my hand
"It's okay," he says, "this will tell you
    where you are"

His unexpected acknowledgment of my
    existence startles me
He smiles
I want to thank him but I cannot speak
I want to cling to him but I cannot move
Still his thoughtful gesture is mine to
    keep
The ambulance door flies open
My gurney slides out and rolls into a
    squat warehouse-like building

The Twilight Zone

Bright lights
Laughter
Chatter
Music
Everyone eating cake

Cries and screams seep through the
    joviality
Tied to a bed near my gurney an old
    man cries out ,"Help! Help! Help me
    please!"
Nobody pays any attention
The lights and bizarre commotion are
    unbearable
I think my head will explode
My blinded eyes search desperately for
    the "kind man"
I want him to take me away from this
    place
But he's eating cake and doesn't hear my
    plea

I'm rolled into a small, three-bed room
The first woman we pass screams threats

"My husband is going to shoot you!
    Shoot you dead!"
The second woman beats a telephone
    against her headboard
I'm rolled onto the third bed and curl up
    terrified
A nurse whips the drape around my bed
"Don't worry about Mary and Rose," she
    says, "They're harmless...however, it's
    a good idea to keep your drape drawn"

After that comforting advice she turns
    out the light and leaves

Mary continues to threaten
Rose weeps and bangs her telephone
    against the wall
My head whirls
My heart thumps like a sledge-hammer

Jaki's words drift back
Something about "moving"
Did she send me here?
No! She wouldn't have
Or...
No. No. No. She is my friend
But then...
Something strange has happened to me

I'm somehow different
"Of course you're different...you're dead,"
    I remind myself

I want to scream like everyone else
Scream! Scream! Scream!
But the act of screaming convulses my
    throat like vomit
Chokes me like vomit
I don't scream
I don't vomit
Instead I lie silent and still on the strange
    bed
Washed over by confusion and fear
I'm not used to fear
I know something's wrong
And fear has taken hold in place of
    understanding

Who abducted me in the middle of the
    night?
Why have I been left in this terrible place
    - a place where desperate people cling
    to life?
Life which is just as desperate to slip
    away
The terror of it is too much

I open my mouth to scream
Nothing comes out
And if it did, who would pay it heed?
I tremble until my teeth chatter

Stay calm

Stay quiet

Breathe deep and stretch tall

Slowly I get a grip on myself

Half of me still wants to scream
The other half fears Mary who's ready
    for battle
I wish I knew whether or not she's
    ambulatory

Exhaustion, denying further thought,
    delivers troubled sleep
I wake in the night, still trapped within
    the twilight zone
It isn't a nightmare it's reality

This strange place is unnervingly quiet
Only a few, far off sobs and muffled
    cries intercept my roommates' snores

Clutched in my hand is the note from
    the "kind man"
The answer to the enigma haunts me
But I don't have my glasses and it's too
    dark to read

A shadow reflects on a curtain near my
    bed
I draw it aside
A window!
A window offering a broken latch!

Freedom!

I ease it open
Fresh air intoxicates me
Stay calm
Stay quiet
Think!
Tonight is not the night
With only a hospital gown to cover me
    and not a clue as to my whereabouts
This is not the night to flee the twilight
    zone

I stare through the grimy window to my
    friend the moon
What has happened to her?

Last night she hung full and bright
Last night when my head was filled with
     colored labels
But tonight she is barely a sliver
What has happened to the moon
     and to me?

It's a mystery
But now I know I have a window
And it's mine!
My secret

I don't believe I'm dead after all

But where am I?

That is the question

Answers? Think Again!

The brazen desert sun bursts over the
  mountains, licks at the drape on my
  window, laughs at the squalor of the
  room that the benevolent light of the
  moon failed to display
The sun also brings light - light to help
  me read
My eyes strain
It's impossible to read the note
The man has written it in a peculiar code
Why a code?
Of course...this is the twilight zone
But is it?
While I don't recognize this place there
  doesn't seem to be anything bizarre
  about it
Just snores from nearby beds and
  housekeeping clatter in the hallway
  beyond
But who brought me here and why?
Have I been in an accident?
I check my body parts
They're all where they should be
I gingerly get out of bed

Nothing hurts although my muscles feel
weak

So the problem must be my head but that
doesn't hurt either

Did I have another horse-riding accident?

Wait a minute! I haven't ridden a horse
in years!

Everything remains a mystery

I clean up as best I can in the small sink,
make my bed then sit on it since it's
the only furniture in the room

I listen to Mary and Rose snore and wait

And wait

And wait

For what I do not know

A doctor and nurse arrive

Answers at last!

"What's your name," the nurse demands

My mouth works frantically to speak

Why am I struggling to say my name?

The nurse is impatient

"What's the day and date," she snaps

I haven't a clue

But confident I can write my name even
if I can't say it, I motion for pencil
and paper

Poised to write I stop short

Words confuse me

Writing my very own name confuses me
Refusing to accept defeat I struggle
    desperately
Something is written but I don't know
    what
The doctor and nurse stare at it
The doctor mutters, "Aphasia"
Aphasia? That's not my name!
The doctor and nurse start to move away
"Wait a minute!" I shriek scrambling
    toward them
"I'm not Aph...Aph...whatever you called
    me. I'm Megan Timothy and I want
    to know why i'm here"
But my words don't come out like I want
    them to
Instead that darned chicken shows up
Startled, both doctor and nurse back
    away in alarm
My instinct tells me to back off, too
I retreat to the far end of the bed, sit still
    and watch
My words disappear into my head where
    they scream only to me
"I don't want to swear or call you
    names...I just want to know where I
    am and why I'm here...please!
    Please!"

Satisfied I'm passive and silent they
show no further interest
This isn't the twilight zone
It's "The Cuckoo's Nest"
And I've just met Nurse Ratchett teamed
up with Doctor No
I feel more sorry for them than for myself
It's easier to repair a broken body than to
repair a callous heart
What has made them lose their
compassion - their desire to heal?
How can they treat another human being
like a vegetable?
Here, right before their eyes is a person
drowning in fear and confusion who,
to them, is nothing but a potato
I sit on my bed and cry
And cry
I can't make sense out of anything
I must get away from this place
But, too exhausted to move, I collapse back
into restless sleep

A resounding clatter in the hallway
rockets me back to life

The curtain around my bed is flung
aside revealing an aggressive herd of
inmates poised to attack the nurses
Rose and Mary burst back to life yelling
like banshees

It's feeding time at the zoo and everyone's
eager to be first in line
A nurse hands me my share - a glass of
water and a cup of pills
Drugs?
I'm suspicious
Why do I need drugs?
The nurse insists
I hold my ground
Rose is more than eager to help me out

Suddenly Jaki is standing at the foot of
my bed
She and the nurse talk, but so fast I can't
follow
Jaki hands me the pills
Because I trust her I take them
She sits on my bed
I stare at her, afraid to blink in case she
evaporates
Oh, please, please don't let her be an
illusion!

"Do you remember what happened to
     you?" she asks

I shake my head

"You have suffered an AVM," she says

More big words I don't understand

"It's a kind of stroke"

A stroke! Me?

How could a super fit, healthy person like
     me have a stroke?

I stare at her in shock and disbelief

"Do you understand?" she asks

"A stroke?" I manage without interference
     from the chicken

I don't like the worried expression on
     Jaki's face

"You were in Moreno Valley Hospital for
     two weeks…"

"Two weeks! What two weeks? And where
     is Moreno Valley?" I ask myself

"…before they sent you here for
     rehabilitation."

"Why do I need to be rehabilitated?" I
     wonder

"You've had some loss of cognitive
     thought and the ability to speak,
     read, and write as a result of brain
     damage."

My head, jumbled with words, can't keep
    up
I start to cry again
Jaki's silent for a while then tells me I'm
    going to be okay
But from her worried expression I don't
    believe her
Before she leaves she assures me that
    either she or Sue will come to see me
    every day
And then she's gone
I don't know whether or not she was really
    here
I cry

I seem to be crying a lot

Thinking Things Over

The nighttime concert tunes up - a
    Wagnerian opera combined with the
    Rolling Stones
Divas, Mary and Rose, howl to beat the
    band
How is it possible to keep my sanity for
    another night?
A nurse finds me huddled on my bed with
    my hands over my ears and offers a
    sleeping pill
Are you kidding? I'm trying to sort out
    my brain not drug it
But as the racket continues I begin to
    wonder if it isn't a good idea
No!
No! No! No! It isn't!

I try hypnosis which has helped me for
    years
But my mind is so disconnected it won't
    concentrate
The only thing left is to join the circus
I scream with the best of them
When it's all over I weep
It is a dangerous thing to allow yourself
    to be seduced by such madness
I open my window, breathe in the fresh
    air, and struggle with the urge to
    flee

Oh, how I long for the serenity of my
    home and Coon Cat curled up next to
    me
I want to remember and understand
    everything Jaki said
Or do I?
The information clamors through my
    battered brain
Stroke...a kind of stroke...brain damage
I'm terrified and confused
What did she mean by "brain damage"?
I have no pain, no wound, no blood I can
    see
Just a little confusion and that always
    passes
At least it always did after the riding
    accidents I had

And then there's the other thing she
    brought up - the question of money
I didn't have much, but now I have none
It's all gone
That's why I'm here at this horror they
    call a rehabilitation center
My situation has reduced me to being a
    ward of the state

My mother died two months ago
Her last years required round-the-clock-
    attention
Not able to work, my funds dwindled
    leaving no possibility of health
    insurance
Soon after Mum died I rented a cottage
    on Jaki's ranch

Before I had time to unpack I was loaded
    onto the ambulance

My life is a fine mess

But at least my friends know where I am
And I have some answers
Any answers are better than none
My brain is frazzled, yes, but I can
    think!
And I do understand...well, mostly

My body is in good working order
But it's essential for my mind to have
    peace and quiet to pull itself
    together
I won't get it here
Where do I go?

I can't expect friends to take
    responsibility for me
It's up to me to make a plan to leave
    this place

Recent events have offered no time to
    mourn my mother
But in my heart lie the gifts she left
    me
Gifts of courage, determination, and will
These are the things that will see me
    through

Getting Organized

It's a new day! I'm alive!
There's no time to waste feeling sorry
  for myself.
I need to fix what I can and figure out
  how to handle the rest.
But first, I need a bath - badly.
Early morning reconnaissance locates a
  shower of sorts.
Actually, it's more like a sheep dip -
  the kind farm animals are herded into
  and hosed down in.
A passing nurse whispers in my ear, "Be
  sure to wear sandals and put towels
  on the floor."
I understand why she wrinkles her nose.
The place is filthy.
I have no sandals but finding towels is
  easy
There's a great big hamper full of them
  in the hallway.
As I reach out for one, the Towel Warden
  slaps my hand.
Unfortunately my polite effort to explain
  my need goes awry and I tell her to
  go "f.... a chicken".
Embarrassed, I try to apologize which
  only makes my words worse.
"You're not allowed in here without a
  nurse. Get back to your room!" she
  snaps.
I feel six years old.
Since verbalizing a response is out of
  the question I resort to crime.
I manage to appropriate four towels and
  throw in a fresh gown and face cloth
  to boot.

Showered, shampooed, and dressed in a fresh gown, I feel terrific although exhausted.

My new criminal career leaves me with a weird sense of accomplishment.

As I pass Mary she drops her hairbrush and asks me to pick it up. When I do, she thanks me with surprising sweetness. She's not so bad after all.

I really shouldn't be so judgmental. This is a difficult place for everyone.

As I head back to my bed the brush falls again. I pick it up.

Rose giggles as Mary deliberately throws down the brush.

"Pick it up, bitch!" she growls, her expression quite mad.

I retreat to my bed leaving the brush on the floor.

Mary goes berserk frothing at the mouth and screaming. I'm relieved she's not ambulatory.

Nurses rush in to calm her and Rose.

I'm ordered to Ratchett's office.

"I hear you've been causing trouble with your roommates," she accuses. "We don't allow that kind of behavior here."

She's as crazy as Mary and Rose and I believe anyone staying here is likely to join them in their insanity.

Ratchett skims over what appear to be my medical records. "Mm, you were a writer? Well, not anymore, honey. You'll be lucky to be able to say your name. Mmm-um, no family, huh. Looks like you're going to be with us for a long, long time. You'd better learn to respect our rules and behave. Do you understand?"

I'm back to being six years old for the second time today. My resentment escalates but I say nothing. The words I need to fight this battle are locked somewhere inside my head where they dance only for me.

"I won't be here for long and I will write again! And until I can write on paper I will write in my mind. Yes! I will!"

I'm marooned on the empty island of my own mind.

No one, not even my friends, understands that though I cannot communicate, other parts of my brain are waking up. My memory and comprehension are kicking in.

Everything before arriving here remains a blur, I remember everything that has happened since the first moment I arrived here, in this place. Everything!

"Especially your malevolence, Ratchett."

Sue arrives armed with a pot of tea and English biscuits. Biscuits she'll do without in a pinch - tea, never.

I'm elated to see her but of course nothing can be said or done until after tea.

It's wonderful to be engaged in a familiar ritual.

Because my speech is so limited, Sue does the talking while I stick mostly to "yes" and "no" and the odd "chicken".

Jaki suggested Sue bring me some deodorant. I introduce her to the "sheep dip" shower.

Back in the room Sue's confronted with Mary and her hairbrush. Poor Sue! She needs more than a cup of tea to recover from Mary's onslaught.

Being with a friend eases my stress. My words become fluent enough to relate the towel-bandit story. We start to giggle and can't stop.

It's so good to laugh!

I realize Jaki and Sue are making a huge effort to come here so I promise myself not to bring up the bad things.

I want them to keep coming.

Oh, God, how I want them to keep coming!

I couldn't bear it if they didn't, but it must be their choice, not my plea.

When it's time for Sue to leave she showers me with gifts of fresh fruit and we giggle over the bananas which I still insist on calling "chickens".

Suddenly, the humor unexpectedly collapses and tears flood down my cheeks.

Damn!

To keep my mind off sorrow I turn it toward exercise. I need it as much for my weak body as I do for my confused, faltering mind. I feel as if I spent the whole two weeks at Moreno Valley Hospital flat on my back.

The in-house gym offers the same quality facility as the sheep-dip. Its most demanding equipment is a set of walkers.

I'm cut short at the door by an irritable attendant who raps her knuckles on the door sign.

"Keep Out! Can't you read?" she snarls.
I stare at the sign. A mere two words and
I can't make head nor tail of them.
Panic!
It's true! It's really true. The reality
of the fact that I can't read hits
home hard.
Neither bad light nor the fact that I
don't have my glasses can explain why
I can't make sense out of the letters.
They could well be some kind of exotic
code.
Now I understand why they were trying to
make me read the alphabet at Moreno
Valley Hospital.

Is this what Jaki meant by "brain damage"?
I realize I've been following familiar
graphic symbols instead of reading
the words on the signs.
My brain feels like a jigsaw puzzle with
missing pieces. But how can that be?
A brain is a brain, not bits and
pieces. Or is it?
I'm suddenly aware I know nothing about
my brain. It's always just kind of
been there clicking along, behaving
itself.
I rush down the hallway looking at signs,
notices, billboards. I can't decipher
one.

How do you live without words?
How do you reason?
How do you resolve problems?
And how can a heart exist without
literature?

Will all the wonderful emotions of my
existence - the things that make me

human - will they just dissolve from lack of expression? How can they survive locked in a silent mind, unable to share or be shared?
I curl up on my bed totally unnerved.

I have an empty head attached to a working body. Does such a thing still have use?
Or will I be banished to a place like this to merely exist? Will I live out the rest of my life here with Nurse Ratchett, Dr. No, and the rest of these inmates - this place with no road maps guiding us anywhere?

I have always been self-reliant. All my life I've rowed my own boat - literally, a number of times.
Then, without warning, my independence evaporated trapping me in an unfamiliar place with unfamiliar people and an unfamiliar Self.
While my brain receives incoming information, outgoing communication is blocked.
The prison wall is clear glass to me, but to those outside it has no light or sound.

There seem to be no doorways in or out.

eight

Another Day

I'm determined to do better.
No more panicking over missing words.
They're only playing a game of hide-and-
    seek. I see them now and then, here
    and there. My tongue is just not fast
    enough to catch them.

No more tears.
And no more wasting time feeling wretched.
    It sounds like one of those New Year
    resolutions you never keep.
But this is no harebrained caprice.
It's serious stuff.

Jaki startles me. "What are you doing?"
    she asks, alarmed, not expecting to
    find me stuffing contraband blankets
    under my mattress.
I really haven't lost my sanity. I'm merely
    attempting to level my backbreaking
    rag of a mattress. At "The Place",
    the name I've given this disaster they
    have the nerve to call a rehab center,
    one learns quickly to do for oneself.
I have wild expectations that Jaki's come
    to take me home.
Mmmm, my own bed! Coon Cat curled up next
    to me! And quiet! Wonderful quiet!
But it's only a wishful thought that
    quickly evaporates. And I'm too unsure
    of my situation to broach the subject.
What if she tells me I'm too broken to
    mend? That I will have to live here
    for the rest of my life? I'm not strong
    enough right now to face such an
    ordeal.

On the bright side, Jaki's brought me treasures. She has my glasses, a carryall of clothes, sandals, and a brand new electric toothbrush.

But most important, she has brought herself.

I refuse to anticipate either Jaki's or Sue's visits. The disappointment, should they not come, would be too painful to bear.

Jaki's life is so busy I don't know how she fits me in. She manages the ranch alone, takes care of her ailing husband, watches out for her aged mother, and never refuses help to anyone who asks.

Jaki looks at me curiously. "Are you feeling okay?"

"Yes."

"You look kind of flushed." I shrug.

She goes on to inform me that we're going to begin fixing my chaotic reading and speech problems. I remain shattered by yesterday's effort to read, but this is a new day - a better day.

And I have a dear friend at my side.

Jaki opens a magazine, points to a wristwatch, and asks me what it is.

I'm mortified when I can't answer. The word is in my head but refuses to come out.

Jaki closes the magazine, hands it to me, and asks me to point out a wristwatch. I flip the pages and identify a watch without delay. How is it that one part of my brain works and the other doesn't?

She explains that the aneurysm scrambled sections of my brain, scattering them like the contents of an upturned filing cabinet.

"Now it's up to you to pick up the pieces, sort them out, and put them back in order." She smiles. "You've already started."

I stare at her.

"Yes! You have! Look at how many more words you have than 'chicken'."

She's right! Words are starting to pop into place.

At last I have a simple, yet descriptive idea of my problem and how to start solving it. My words just need organization.

I knew they weren't really lost!

I'm very excited. Tidying up a "filing cabinet" doesn't sound that difficult.

Jaki is less cavalier about it. She warns of long days of very hard work. That doesn't scare me. I've never been afraid of hard work.

"If this... er... is only, I mean... um... um... all that... y'know... um... that makes me ill... no! All... that's... wrong... can... I... go... home?"

She demurs. The worried look in her eyes tells me there's more to it. "We have to make sure you can live on your own first," she says.

I want to argue that I can, but I know that when I'm upset the words come out badly and make me look worse than I am.

So I die a little inside and nod reluctant agreement.

But all in all it has been a good day!

My friend has visited and brought me hope.

I have clothes. I don't have to go barefoot in the awful sheep-dip anymore. My bed won't break my back tonight.

And if the worst comes to the worst, I can flee this place without being arrested for indecent exposure.

And...I will soon be able to read directions.

I resist putting my clothes in the drawers. It would put life here on too much of a permanent basis. Instead I keep the packed carryall on top of the night stand.

I must exercise! My weak limbs cry out to regain their former strength. I must be ready should I decide to flee. Right now I wouldn't get farther than a few yards.

I start by walking around the circular inside hallway. It's hard. I'm so weak I teeter around like a drunkard. Ratchett stares at me staggering past her office door.

The sight of the witch inspires me to straighten up, stride out, and complete my mission. I collapse onto my bed exhausted but exhilarated.

I open the magazine Jaki left to work on my reading. While I can visually recognize the pictures their words still remain hidden. I can't make any sense of the letters or sound them out. No words. No letters. Only a constant mystery.

Jaki's right. This is a hard nut to crack.

But then I'm a hard-headed woman!

The Inmates

Even Mary and Rose are quiet this morning.

Mrs. Warfield is dead.

While an inmate's death doesn't generally draw much attention Mrs. Warfield is different. She has endured thirty-six years of purgatory in this Dickensian institution. That kind of stamina and resilience demands respect.

Mrs. Warfield arrived here at age sixty four-and checked out two days before her centennial celebration.

I'm close enough to sixty-four to feel its breath on my neck.

I wonder...

I wonder if Mrs. Warfield, like me, arrived here penniless with no place else to go.

Am I doomed to the same fate? Thirty days, let alone thirty years, is more than I can bear.

My window beckons.

I investigate the other inmates. Many, like me, don't speak much. Is it because they can't? Or, is it some complicated personal decision?

Bill, a young man, shuffles around the hallway all day pushing a homemade walker. He's wrapped in an habitual smile but never utters a word or focuses his eyes.

Nothing stops his endless shuffle to wherever it's taking him - not even tottering into a wall. His determined lock-shuffle keeps marching on the spot until someone straightens him out.

The mysterious Mrs. Trotter appears to be a woman of means. She has a room to herself decorated with her own furniture - good antiques, sumptuous silk drapes, two oriental rugs, a stunning chaise, and a beautiful oak bed.

She's always immaculately dressed and groomed. Catch her eye and she gives a pained smile but never speaks.

I meet Leonard. He speaks long and loud to anyone whether they listen or not.

His bed is surrounded by padlocked bookcases stuffed to the hilt - treasures no one is allowed to touch.

He invites me to watch Jeopardy in the common TV room. The noise and bright flickering of the TV screen instantly drive my head to distraction.

No TV for me!

Mell asks me to push him around in his wheelchair. I'm happy to help out. An enormous bandage wraps his shaved head and his legs appear alarmingly swollen.

At least he speaks.

But Ratchett shows up and accuses me of interfering and scolds Mell for being too lazy to wheel himself.

Not all the staff and nurses are Ratchett-like, but all are grossly over worked among the large population of difficult inmates. They simply do not have time for the Florence Nightingale touch.

My new friend, a housekeeper named Margaret, helps me. Every morning she tells me the day, date, and her name. But, by the time she finishes mopping the floor they have slipped out of my mind.

She goes through it all again before she leaves. I struggle to hold on to the slippery words, but as she disappears so do they. It's new information that won't stick.

Minute details from my past have started to trickle back to the surface of my mind - things that happened as a child decades past. But, I can't remember Margaret's name from a minute ago - that name repeated to me over and over, day after day.

Ratchett's real name also eludes me. I named her "Ratchett" after a movie character I remember from about twenty years ago. It fits and is all I really want to know about the woman.

I like Jose and Sam. Jose composes religious music. Sam creates uplifting greeting cards he illustrates with floral designs.

The world is not lost. There are still people alive who create!

And then there's Viola! Very old, very frail, and once a stunning beauty. She huddles on her wheelchair and weeps.

No one pays her any attention.

Tess is only thirty-two. She appears to be in chronic pain but volunteers no information on how or why. The corner of her room is densely decorated with memorabilia - another life fighting off the encroachment of unwanted change.

Keeping watch with Tess is Nelly, a sad, little parakeet locked in a cage. Neither Nelly nor Tess will ever fly again. Robbed of their liberty, all that's left is to guard fast-fading memories. They've been here too long, their resolve too deeply undermined by the system.

Flight, the greatest gift to us all, has been stolen.

I will never let that happen to me.

Never!

I'm different!

ten

Sue and Jaki

As sure as the sun rises, so do Jaki and Sue keep their word. One or the other comes to see me every day. As eager as I am to see them, it still hurts to have only the tears of a fool and the weakness of a child to offer.

I want to be whole in their eyes. I want to be the reason a smile comes to their faces. I want to be deserving of them.

For a short time each day my wish is granted. The touch of their hands heals my fresh scars and makes me whole again.

But, uncertainty has an insatiable appetite. I fight to control it, afraid my constant needs will swallow them up.

Nothing is said about my coming home. I don't dare ask. Exactly how ill I am and whether or not I have the ability to care for myself remain unanswered questions, ones I need to gather strength to ask. Right now the load I carry wouldn't weigh as much as a feather. To simply survive I must put these questions out of my mind for now.

In the meantime Jaki and Sue work hard to help restore my communicative losses. Intensive as the sessions are, they yield little.

To outsiders my brain is silent. To me it screeches like a giant maul crushing twisted metal. When the hammer

– my tongue - hits the words I've worked so hard to gather, they split and shatter.

Some days I can't bear the thought of this absurd word game. I can't bear to see the pity in my friends' eyes when they think I'm not looking. But I can't afford the luxury of frustration. I have to find my way back to the real world.

Both of my friends show enormous concern for my comfort. One side of me is appreciative, the other, fed with growing paranoia is suspicious.

Sue brings me ear-plugs to help me through the night, fresh fruit so I have something civilized to eat, and a framed picture of us at my recent birthday.

Jaki arrives with a wonderful down mattress cover that transforms the awful bed into something almost luxurious. She also brings me slippers and body lotion. The immediate comfort of these things is wonderful but later, when I'm alone, I see them as a threat - a frightening message that I'm being settled in for keeps.

Truth is, I've been remiss in truly appreciating my friends. Even before this incident they stood by me, supporting me as my mother failed. The three weeks before Mum died, Sue came everyday. She comforted my Mum and taught me to overcome past grievances and to give of myself in a way I had not had the courage to do. I never asked her to come, but she arrived every day and sat with Mum and me for hours.

Now she is doing it again.

I ask Sue if it's my fault my brain exploded, what with my hard-driven life and all the accidents I've had.

She says, "No, an AVM is a birth defect...one of those silent, hidden things you don't know you have until it makes a statement. This can be anytime during your life from birth to old age."

At least mine had the consideration not to manifest itself until my mum passed away.

I feel better that it's not my fault. Even more so since I've discovered something unexpectedly positive.

"Do you... um... I mean... er... have you noticed something different in... um... in... in my speech?"

She gives me a sidelong glance.

"No! Not the... what do you call it? Not the... um... chicken," I insist. "Something... um... else."

"Well, you are rather short on words."

"But... um... listen... listen to the ones I have! I... I mean, I... er... I stumble, yes, but I don't stammer!"

She stares at me blankly.

"That... what is it? What is it? Demon! That demon that's tormented me my whole life has... has disappeared... just disappeared!"

She looks at me, stunned. "You're right! Amazing! And weird'

"It's the... the irony of it that's weird! First... I... I can't speak because I stammer, now... now I can't speak because I've... um... I've lost my words."

We stare at each other then burst out laughing.

Jaki arrives after a run-in with Ratchett over my red face. Ratchett doesn't think there's anything wrong with me and complains I pace up and down the hallway. Jaki assured her I'm just trying to get some exercise. Ratchett declares pacing indicates instability, as does my penchant for black clothing. Jaki explains that in the twenty years she's known me I've mostly worn black clothes. Ratchett insists it's a sign of depression as is my refusal to cooperate with social and therapeutic activities.

Jaki tells me I need to just play the game. "Don't let that old bat have an excuse to say you're crazy."

I shrug.

"Don't complicate things! Sue and I agree you shouldn't be in a place like this. But since we're not family, the state is reluctant to release you to us until you prove yourself capable of making your own decisions and caring for yourself."

Flabbergasted to learn my friends are working to get me out, I immediately agree to play the game.

I'm so moved by what I've learned Jaki and Sue are doing for me my words freeze, unlocking the floodgate of emotion I've fought so hard to control.

I'm swamped in a flood of tears.
    Damn it! Crying again!
    Sue and Jaki are my only rainbows in
this stormy sky.

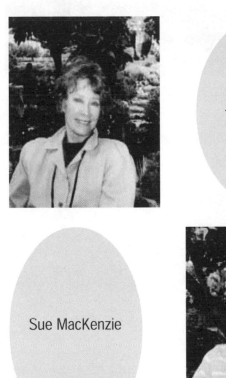

Jaki Markarian

Sue MacKenzie

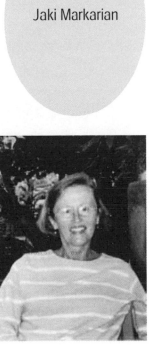

L-R: Megan, Jaki, Sue

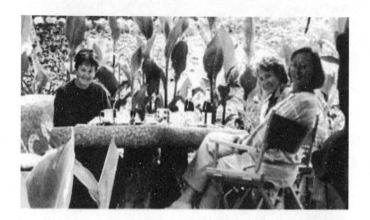

Playing The Game

As I ready myself for "therapeutic activities" a woman of vast girth vibrates my brain whit a strident bellow. "Shower day!"

Shower day? After a week I'm finally offered a sheep dip?

"Let's go! Let's go," she cries.

I decline the offer, relieved to have organized a surreptitious shower system between the night and day shifts. The woman grabs my arms and sniffs my pits. I've passed inspection and she leaves me to recover from yet another round of humiliation.

My first social event is lunch. Conversation is not a pleasant highlight but infernal chatter runs rampant. It bounces from wall to wall, ceiling to floor. I doubt my head will survive the incessant noise.

"Sit anywhere you like," says the harassed attendant. But she's not in charge. The inmates are and they've rigged the rules.

My first faux pas is to sit with Jose and Sam. Instead of lunch, I earn a scarlet letter. The dining room, by inmate rules, is strictly non co-ed. Men line up on one side and women the other.

I try Mrs. Trotter's table next. I should have known better. She sits alone, her table dressed with a spotless damask napkin and an elegant wine glass. She doesn't have to say anything. Her pained expression is enough to send me on my way.

My next try is at a table of three mild looking ladies. Suddenly, a forth woman appears dressed for battle, makeup equal to war paint and a deadly handbag poised for attack.

"Sorry Jaki, I'm eating in my room."

Social Activities are intended to prepare us for life on the "outside". There's dancing in the style of one hand clapping. I'm the only one with two functioning legs. Everyone else is either severely incapacitated or mute or both.

Another event involves eating ice cream, the point of which, as therapy, evades me. Nevertheless, it draws a record crowd.

There's also a sing-along led by the Activities Director. Her loud guitar and even louder voice sends my head into spasms and I'm done for.

The agenda also includes finger painting. I'm inspired!

Out of no where comes the letter "Y". I proceed to create a bold, bright series of the ever lasting "why?!".

The Activities Director doesn't get it and suggests I'd do better if I stuck to pretty daises. I acquiesce, but it causes a riot when I convince the others it would be fun to paint daisies on each others' faces.

Every one with a semblance of a

working brain shows up for Bingo. I hate Bingo! The Activities Director seats me next to her. Obviously it's considered wise to keep an eye on someone who paints "Y"s.

The game starts with a lot of loud noise. I'm searching for a way out when someone yells "Five!" The director bangs on my sheet yelling "Five! Five! Five!" I search but numbers jumble in my head worse than letters. Next thing I know the Director slams a dollar bill on my sheet. "Hooray! You've won!" she shouts.

I'm furious. First humiliated, now patronized, I slide the dollar back in front of her. She slides it back to me. We battle until the reality of the dollar sinks in. It's money! And I'm going to need money to flee this place.

I can't remember how much a dollar is worth or just what it will buy, but who cares. It's money. I snatch it back, stuff it down my front, and watch for more, steeling my throbbing head against the noise.

The next day when the mute-and-lame are rolled in I figure I'm in trouble. We're seated in a circle wearing team caps of blue and red and are encouraged to throw soft pillow balls at each other.

I regress, not just to a five-year-old but all the way back to a two-year-old.

Enough!

I throw down my cap.

"No, dear...throw the ball not the cap!"

I head for the door rather than strangling her.

"Come back, sweetheart, were not finished."

"Dear" and "sweetheart" in one breath!

A number of the mute-and-lame watch me intently. My god! They're alive! They understand! Just like me, they're locked inside their heads.

I fold my arms defiantly and watch them. They follow. I'm shocked and outraged. How much do these people understand? How long have they been left here to flounder? If it weren't for Jaki and Sue I could be joining them permanently.

"Teach us!" I growl. "Don't... don't um... in...insult us! We're not stupid! We're um... we're human like you, just lost....just..." I'm so incensed my words cave in and the f...ing chicken returns with a vengeance.

What's the use?

As I stride out I hear tentative applause - a "thank you" from some of the silent people for my small rebellion. It moves me to tears. Until this moment I too thought of them as being nothing of consequence. But looking hard, I see from the inside. I see through their eyes what they see.

It is they who are the courageous ones, not me. I raise a clenched fist in their honor.

Protective of my sanity I refuse to engage in the farce they call "therapeutic activity". Ratchett jumps all over me. I keep my eyes to the floor. I dare not look at her or open my ears to her. I'm too close to wringing off her neck.

Instead I talk to her inside my head. *"To you I'm nothing but a cash cow churning out taxpayer dollars for your zoo. But you're wrong! I'm very much alive inside. I still dream with my eyes wide open. My soul still holds together laughter, passion, joy - and yes, sadness and fear - and for you right now, a lot of anger. My dreams and I live. You, you sad excuse for a human, dream only at night. Nighttime dreams are only illusions. They lie lifeless in eyes closed shut. And you lie lifeless within them."*

Jaki shows up. "Ratchett's complaining that you're refusing therapy."

"I'm not going back to... er... back..."

"Megan, you know we have to keep Ratchett happy right now. Besides, it's essential you continue with speech therapy."

"Speech therapy? You mean with you... and... um... and Sue?"

"No, the speech therapy the state is paying for you to have twice a day." Her voice has an edge to it I'm not used to hearing.

"I only... er... er speak... no! I mean read? I only read with you... um...

you and Sue."

"No, you have..."

"Only you and Sue!"

I get so mad when people, even my friends, think I'm stupid just because I can't speak!

"Only me and Sue?" Jaki repeats, starting to understand what I'm telling her.

"I need to learn! Not play.... um... um... what is it children do? Play games... games! Or... shit! Shit! Shit!" I'm taking to milder expletives now when my words run amuck.

"Games as in cards, ping-pong... children's games?" Jaki asks.

I nod vigorously.

"No speech or reading therapy?"

When is she going to believe me! I shake my head.

Jaki turns white with anger and strides off to confront Ratchett.

twelve

Therapy

Evening brings a speech therapist, a wan-looking woman who wastes no time on niceties or introduction. She goes straight to work scrawling Post-it labels and sticking them on my bed, the wall, light, toilet door, and window.

"Read!" she commands, collapsing on the chair she dragged in.

"Read? If I could I wouldn't need you," I snap silently, staring at her.

She sighs heavily, sits up and raps sharply on the footboard. "Bed!" she blares out as if I were deaf.

Like the parrot I've become I immediately imitate her.

She leads me by the nose through the rest of the yellow Post-its. I'm so fed-up being an incoherent, inarticulate mess tears flow down my cheeks. Another excuse to cry. I'm pretty fed-up with that, too.

The therapist leans back on her chair, shuts her eyes, and appears to fall asleep.

Although I have no experience in therapy, I can see this woman is not going to be of any help to me. There is no sense of communication, information, or knowledge. But so desperate am I for help I'll speak to anyone, even someone who's asleep.

Whispering softly, I struggle for words as best I can. I tell her about the frustration and fear of not being able to communicate, the stress of being cooped up with Mary and Rose, and my greatest fear, that my friends will tire of the effort it's taking to sort me out.

I must have somehow managed an eloquent speech for when she opens her eyes she is a very different person. She introduces herself. Her name is Ann and she becomes my ally.

The morning speech therapy session is much worse. Ann can't come so my therapy is handed over to a giddy young girl whose regular job is pushing wheelchairs. She leads me around, vaguely pointing out familiar objects and giggling when I can't name them.

Other giggly interns join in. It's fun to train a monkey!

The humiliation is such agony I can barely contain my rage.

As friendly as Ann has become, her therapy doesn't improve. I make less progress with her than I do with Sue and Jaki. Out of the two dozen simple objects illustrated on the pages Ann shows me, I'm only able to verbally identify one – cigarette.

It continues to be the same old thing. If asked to point out a verbalized item I have no problem. It's reading independently and retaining words just learned that's impossible for me. No one so far seems to have any understanding of my problem.

Or does it mean that part of my brain

has been destroyed?

The more I try to eject this cold, hard thought, the tighter it embraces me. I'm terrified. My confidence, which has always seen me through the toughest situation, is steadily being shredded by this place and its inherent insanity.

Meanwhile, Jaki's at war with Ratchett who declares I'd rather pace idly around the hall than make an effort to read.

I need information, dammit! Clear, concise words uncluttered with medical jargon. I want to ask questions but the words won't come out. I want to read books to gather answers but I can't even get through the funny pages right now.

I'm trying to hold on but I feel myself slipping. I think I'm going mad and I never want to hear the word "therapy" again!

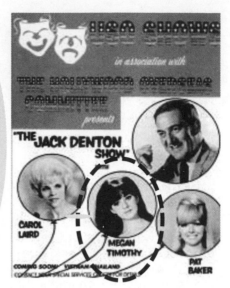

Megan toured S.E. Asia as a singer with the Jack Denton Show during the Vietnam War.

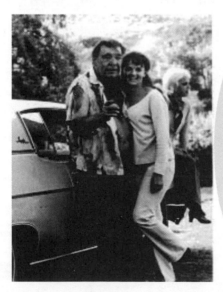

In 1969, Megan (R) starred with Lon Chaney (L) in the movie, "A Time To Run".

thirteen

A Christian Woman

Ann wins her battle to have me moved. No more raucous roommates. In fact, the new one is silent save for her soft, rhythmic respirator air tube and an odd fart. Before I have time to adjust to my comatose companion, someone else dies, freeing up a less eerie room.

I meet Mable.

The constant unnerving flow of souls passing through "The Place" convinces Mable that her call is imminent. Determined to arrive with all her ducks in a row on Judgment Day, she devotes her time to memorizing the entire Bible.

"If you don't have all the right answers, you'll be forbidden to enter the gates of Heaven. Are you ready?" she whispers.

I explain as best I can that I'm having enough trouble with basic English without attempting Biblical tests. Convinced I'm doomed, she promises to pray for my condemned soul.

Mable's family is less sympathetic. There's no doubt in their minds that I am sin personified. "God only strikes down those who are deserving of His wrath," they mutter as if I'm unable to hear or understand. "For her to have been struck dumb proves what an evil mind hers must have been." Judgment is passed, any defense considered irrelevant.

Night is the worst time for Mable. At sundown she disappears under a voluminous big-hair wig — camouflage to ward off the probing eyes of the devil and his troops of vampires searching for fuel to feed their hell-fire.

"Listen," she hisses, "They're calling them."

"Who's calling what?" I ask.

"Them! Them!" she breathes, jerking her head toward the nightly wailing dirge, "They're telling them which of us to take."

"Why don't you put in a word to God for help?" I suggest.

My ignorance stuns her. "Sinners who can't recite the Bible have no hope of being saved. My brother says I still make too many mistakes." She bursts into tears. Oh, dear! I really think I may have been too hasty in forsaking the relative peace offered by the comatose companion.

In an attempt to cheer Mable up in the morning, I share the beautiful bouquet of yellow roses sent to me by my literary agent, Lisa FitzGerald. The flowers morph Mable into a completely different person. Her former profession as a florist now shows itself in her care for these lovely flowers.

Thoughts of death and the devil fly out of the window the moment I suggest she arrange the roses. Her eyes light up. She becomes authoritative and orders me to find a vase and to bring water, scissors, and newspaper. She even encourages me to climb out the window to gather filler greenery from the pathetic landscaping brushes. The only time I ever see her laugh is when my pants catch on a nail, trapping me on the window-sill. Her arrangement is stunning and I tell her it would be selfish to keep it to ourselves. She agrees.

"But," I add, "if we move the flowers to the lobby you'll have to supervise."

She's nervous. Mable can't remember when she last left her bed.

I borrow Viola's wheelchair and a nurse helps Mable into it. Life flows into her. She's a different person. Mable has a purpose — a mission...that is until her family arrives to find her consorting with the very heathen who just might be the devil himself. There's Hell to pay. I'm in trouble and Mable topples.

Again, I'm overwhelmed by the enormity of life and death - the two great gifts we all are given but seldom comprehend. We are alone on this journey. There are no teachers, no pupils, no books, no gurus to guide us. In the end we each have to find our own way through the maze.

Embrace it! Celebrate it! Life and death, our only true possessions, paradoxically, are not ours to choose. However, open hearts and open minds help free us to find our bearings.

Neither life nor death can be adequately explained by words. Both stamp us with knowledge we understand yet cannot express. But, because we have this unspoken knowledge we're able to embrace them both without fear, if we choose to.

Fear comes only when we lose courage and allow others to direct and lead us on this, our most personal journey.

Megan hiked the Grand Canyon and rafted down the Colorado - just another adventure for this indominable woman!

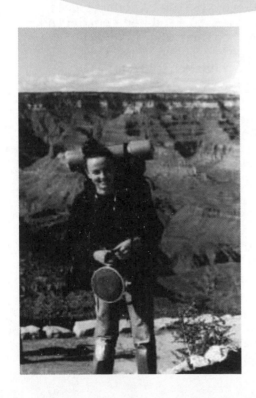

fourteen

Fear Of Flying

"We've done it!" Sue exclaims, too excited to pour her tea. "Jaki's taking you home tomorrow!"

I can't believe it! Home? I'm going home!

Sue complains that I never come to see her off when she leaves. "Come out to the car," she says when we reach the front door.

Out to the car? Outside? The idea unnerves me.

"Come on, a little walk will do you good."

I resist.

Sue insists. Ignoring my discomfort she leads me firmly by the hand to the neighboring school playground. I'm almost a basket case. What's happened to this person who biked solo around half the world, hiked the Macho Pichu Trail alone, rafted down the Mississippi - not to mention the Amazon and the Colorado Rivers?

I suddenly realize why the window locks haven't been fixed. There's no need for them. What holds people here are not locks and bars but something invisible and far more powerful - hopelessness, despair, paranoia, and dissociation of personality.

And I was arrogant enough to believe I was different - stronger and smarter than anyone else.

My grand plan to escape out of my window may have been serious that first night, but after that nothing more than a farce. I fizzled under pressure that left nothing but the blinding dust of bravado.

After only two weeks I dodder on the very edge of becoming Tess, Nelly, and all the others I scorn. How long before my wings, like theirs, are truly clipped and I never fly again? These wings, fabricated by humor, support a mind molded from laughter. And that is the very breath of life.

I walk the school playground with Sue struggling to replace oppression with giddy laughter. It doesn't matter how silly I get now as long as I laugh enough to spread my snared wings and breathe.

fifteen

Viola

Jaki arrives to take me home. Margaret, the housekeeper, gives me a notebook and a set of pencils to help me start writing again.

Sam has made me one of his special cards.

Jose's composed a hymn to keep me safe on my journey.

Mable prays for my lost soul.

I've said goodbye to everyone I care about except Viola.

"Goodbye" - a cold, hard word. And not one that Viola deserves. I don't want to think about her. I don't have to. She's merely a fragment of the dark life I'm leaving behind - a shadowy reflection of two confused weeks.

Lies!

Viola has come to mean more to me than that. And she holds me to it, dancing across my mind like a dragonfly over water, reflecting images of the first time I saw her so lost and alone, curled up in her wheelchair weeping.

"Don't worry about her", the nurse had said. "That's all she ever does. She cries."

This lovely face without a name, stripped of sunshine on its cheeks, has become my obsession.

Our lives gradually meld. At first she gave me nothing but her tears. I gave her songs. She didn't mind my frazzled brain making up the music. I took her for walks around the building when Ratchett wasn't looking. We visited the sparrows near the front door and fed them crumbs from our food trays. The birds revived Viola's smile, gave her back the grace to raise her hands in greeting.

Like manna from a benevolent God, somewhere everyday I found a flower to put in her hair. And the lobby mirror showed her how beautiful she looked.

Yesterday, for the first time, she took my hand and pressed it to her cheek.

It was my turn to weep.

How can I abandon Viola?

Jaki's ready to leave.

I mutter about forgetting something and hurry down the hallway. Viola's room is empty, her bed stripped. Her much loved little pink and yellow afghan is gone. Shadows no longer hide the sunshine from her face.

She's come full circle, earned her wings and flown. And in doing so allows me to spread mine.

sixteen

Heading Home

I've despised "The Place" since the moment I arrived - strove to leave it, fought to escape it. But now, as the car moves onto the freeway, I vacillate. The real world has grown tall and wide and appears no longer friendly or familiar. The freeway stretches out a frightening distance and is traveled by hundreds of cars speeding along. The boisterous traffic chants mockingly in a voice eerily reminiscent of Ratchett's guttural tone.

"You'll be back! You'll be back! You'll be back!" it seems to sing.

I shudder. Anger and fear mix and boil within, not against Ratchett or this wild new world, but against myself.

Who is this fragile person wracked with doubt and confusion?

I may look the same but I'm not.

I don't know who I am. I hardly remember who I was.

Jaki talks to me but I barely hear her.

I want to go back to "The Place". I don't care if Ratchett leers or the opera howls all night. I want to be where things are familiar, and that means "The Place." That has become my reality.

But is it reality or actually a mirage?

I'm so confused.

The voice imprisoned in my head shouts, *"I am your reality, your real voice, listen to me! I will find my way back to you. You won't always have to live with a stranger. I promise!"*

"Home." Another unnervingly foreign place.

My disorganized belongings lie as scattered as my disorganized brain. Stacks of moving boxes neatly labeled with words I cannot read are piled here and there. Just as the strangeness of it begins to incite panic, Coon Cat appears, welcoming me with a voice I know and love. It starts to feel like "home."

I feel much better when I see the familiar sheets and blankets on the bed and sense the comfort of my very own mattress. Jaki leaves me to rest.

Other welcoming voices call out. The old donkey brays, a rooster crows, far-off dogs bark, and a horse whinnies.

At last I feel safe and loved.

I'm on my way back to the world I know.

I am home

Finally, with Coon Cat curled up beside me, peace rocks me into glorious sleep - the first tranquil sleep after a month of utter chaos.

seventeen

Coming Alive!

I wake to hear Coon Cat purring in my ear. Energy, strength and hope flow through me washing away the debris of fear and anxiety. I'm on a new journey with an old friend - myself .

Cleansed of the slime from that dark cave, I need to stretch out and live a little, push myself to my new limits, and learn to trust myself a whole lot. I revel in my hard-earned freedom.

The air is clean. The sky goes on forever and ever. My old self is gratified. Together we join hands and the horrors of "The Place" begin to fade. I feel safe in this small house beside Jaki's bigger one.

Jaki presents me with a big box of children's reading materials donated by a retired schoolteacher friend. It's the big, basic alphabet book that grabs my attention. Lots of bright, colorful letters and numbers, skilled pilots ready to guide me out of the darkness that took over my head. Jaki comes over every night after her chores to help me read.

It's late October and the desert nights turn in early, wrapped tightly in a sharp chill. It's inconsequential to us that the house has no heat. Jaki's going through hot flashes and my head feels better when chilled like a bottle of white wine.

Sue, a woman who appreciates comfort, thinks we've both lost our minds.

Jaki remains apprehensive about my state of health. Who can blame her? My brain is a crap-shoot right now. It may explode again any minute or it may never suffer another "incident" for the rest of my life. No one knows. The uncertainty is nerve-wracking to both me and my friends.

To help control the risk of having further aneurysms I must continue taking the anti-seizure medication three times a day. It may be protecting me on one hand but on the other it leaves me looking as flushed as an excited tom-turkey. And since the state continues to drag its feet regarding my MediCal approval I can't have it checked, yet.

I appreciate Jaki's courage in bringing me back to the ranch in my precarious condition and will gladly cooperate with her scheme to keep me safe. My friend, Myriam, rushes a Fedex package of electronic gadgets from Los Angeles. It contains everything from walkie-talkies to beepers to something that reminds me of a house arrest ankle bracelet. The get-up makes it possible to monitor my whereabouts anywhere on the ranch and for me to call for help should I need it.

But there's a problem. The gadgets are operated by pressing letters and numbers. As simple as they are, they prove too complex for me.

Secretly I'm relieved not to be trussed up. However, I do have some luck mastering the wireless telephone after several intense days of practice. But, because I'm still so easily confused, we initially limit the phone to just two numbers, Jaki's and Sue's.

Sue introduces me to the local supermarket. While I'm unable to read or verbalize names of items, I do recognize them visually which enables me to shop. Except for yogurt. Locating the brand I like is easy. Determining whether it's "Fruit on the Bottom" or "Pre-stirred" is my dilemma. The labels are identical, only the words classify which kind they are. I'm stumped. The real world lurks with pitfalls I never anticipated.

Both Sue and Jaki decide I need to socialize. Using her formidable put-together skills Jaki styles my hair, does my makeup, and dresses me in a stunning black outfit of hers. We arrive at her friend Elena's party where I'm overcome by an uncontrollable urge to tell everyone about my AVM, my mother's death, and the horrors of "The Place".

Cornering a man I've never met, my words tumble forth slurred and jarred and sliding out of control like those of a drunk. The more the poor man's eyes glaze over, the more determined I am to tell my story. I must tell it and he must listen! The whole world has to be made aware of my tsunami-like crisis. I can't stop and it's impossible to tell whether I'm blushing out of embarrassment or an attack of the anti-seizure drug.

The unfortunate man escapes my clutches when Elena gathers us all to move to the Hemet Mall for the Annual Autumn Elegance Party. The mall, bright and loud, sets off both panic and the urge to scream out my story. I desperately need Jaki's help but my words have become so muddled it's impossible to communicate. Instead, I stuff my mouth with copious amounts of cheesecake in an effort to stop myself from babbling. Soon, I'm too nauseous to bother about enlightening the world with my personal drama.

The past several days have made me aware I'm not quite ready for primetime!

I long, more than ever, to be able to talk to someone. But I can't. My speech is still far too elemental to succeed in discussion of any depth. And, so I'm limited to speaking to myself. Within my head my thoughts and words are clear, the muddled mess that pours out of my mouth definitely is not.

I know I won't succeed in my endeavor to improve until I allow the time and patience this hard job ahead of me demands. To be patient is to calmly endure. And allowing time means working toward a goal without imposing an aritificial time limit.

I come to realize that patience is not a commodity to be bartered - it's a process that must be honored.

The System

Jaki's still fighting to get me into Moreno Valley State Hospital for a check up on the effects the anti-seizure medication is having on me. But alas, I've still not been accepted by MediCal and have no money to pay for a visit. I'm stuck hovering in the no-man's-land otherwise known as MediCal-Pending. And my status will remain "pending" until I'm proven penniless which is far more difficult than you can ever imagine.

It takes an enormous amount of time, patience and paper work to prove you're poor in America. It's a dirty word no one wants to face.

Jaki has a briefcase stuffed with "proof" but it's not enough. It's never enough. The inquisitionists Sacramento has lined up at the hospital to interrogate us deadbeats continue to demand more. They hunger for paperwork like a pack of starving wolves.

If you press your pathetic face to the window often enough they may reluctantly grant limited MediCal-Pending vouchers, but only if the Luck Gods are smiling on you.

Among the three of us we manage to round up a voucher, but it doesn't come cheap. It has to be renewed regularly through a Byzantine system that requires a 5:00 AM lineup. Arrive one minute later than 5:00 and you're out of luck - the daily quota of numbers that only give you the right to stand in line, will be gone. Hordes of indigents seem to camp overnight to assure their place in line.

We start off before dawn on the two-hour drive to the hospital. Even though I now have an authorized MediCal-Pending voucher I still have to line up again for a daily "blue card" before anyone will look at me. So many cards, approvals, stamps, phone calls, computer validations, face to face interrogations. How on earth the much-publicized "MediCal fraud" ever gets into the California state heath system is a mystery. Fort Knox isn't this well guarded.

I fuss and fret over the time all this takes out of my friends' lives. I could possibly make it by bus even though the bus stop is seven miles from the ranch. But I would never survive the hospital bureaucracy without an advocate representing my interests. Sue insists I learn to accept help and accept it with grace. "If it were the other way round you'd do the same for us," she says. I honestly don't know if I'm that good a person and that's what chafes the most.

Moreno Valley Hospital is a totally foreign place to me. Sue and Jaki can't believe I have no recollection of my two-week stay there. "Recollection or not," Sue says, "Prepare to make a lot of apologies. You raised hell..."

"What hell?"

"Well, you were...um...difficult," Jaki adds tactfully.

Sue snorts. "You yelled, swore like a trooper, and dedicated special malice toward anyone with a bedpan."

"Well, I hate those things."

"The loads of medical equipment attached to you restricted you to your bed but you were not having any of it and fought like a maniac to get to the bathroom."

Jaki, nods in agreement, adding, "And you became so determined to go home they had to place a guard at your bed."

I don't believe either of them. After all, they are known to joke around. However, to save my ribs from Sue's demanding nudges, I trot out apologies for unremembered grievances delivered to unknown persons. Their forgiving expressions tell me there must be something in it after all.

By the time we get to Dr. K, the brain surgeon, I've got my act down pat. But she's so concerned about my red face she doesn't give me a chance to perform. "Why did you take so long to have this seen?" she scolds.

None of us have the energy to explain the MediCal nightmare. I'm just relieved to have the problem solved. She immediately hands us a new anti-seizure prescription and tells her nurse to make sure I have another check up the following week.

Dr. K stares at me for a moment. "Your brain," she says, "has suffered severe trauma which will take about a year to stabilize. Until then we cannot commence with treatment."

"But the prognosis...?" Sue asks anxiously.

"Knowledge and treatment of the brain, the most complex of organs, is growing rapidly," Dr. K replies confidently. "We'll consider all the opportunities at the end of the year and in the meantime you must continue with the medication, avoid lifting heavy weights, throwing up, strenuous bowel movements or anything that puts pressure on the brain. And NO aspirin!"

I learn then that aspirin, and indeed, any anti-inflammatory drugs are disastrous for anyone in my condition. Simple aspirin - the only drug I've ever taken - turns out to be my nemesis.

In 1999, during a solo eight-month, ten-thousand mile bike trip, I was sometimes taking six aspirins a day for pain that I diagnosed as stress, sciatica, or just normal aches born of physical exhaustion. Even though these pains were not headaches, I was later told, they could well have been warning signs of the impending AVM. But on the back roads of places like Morocco, Turkey, and the Balkans, pain relievers other than aspirin did not exist. Besides, I felt so confident using something as benign as aspirin. It's a miracle I survived that trip with my ripening AVM.

My friends and I are unusually quiet as we head down to the Speech Therapy Department. We'd all been hoping for Dr. K to deliver a silver bullet, not a vague uncertain waiting game.

"Hello!" says a cheery voice behind us. Of course Jaki and Sue recognize Ms. X but I don't. As I prepare to trot out my customary apology, she stands back, takes a good look at me, and says "You did well at the rehabilitation center...I didn't expect you'd be out so soon."

I freeze. "You sent me?"

"Yes."

"Why?"

"Well, we had to get you all better now, didn't we?"

I'm astonished! Ms. X is proud of herself. She acts as if she checked me into a four-star resort not a Devil's Island hell-hole. My blazing tongue-lashing is curbed when my jaw freezes. But my arms and hands aren't locked so why not just wring her neck instead? I eyeball her with the ferocious stare I learned from a maniacal great aunt and step forward.

Startled, she backs away. Ah! The wild eyes scare her. Good! On second thought scaring her might be a better idea rather than wringing her neck. At least it'll get me in less trouble than homicide. I take another step. She backs into the elevator door. This is fun! I figure Ms. X owes me whatever sick sort of fun pleases me.

I hear Sue's unusually nervous voice. "Megan, are you alright?"

I must be doing a good job if I'm scaring my

friends. The elevator door opens and Ms. X almost falls in backwards scattering the sheaf of papers she has in her hands. The door slides shut and she disappears. I'm about to throw my head back laughing when I hear Sue's reprimand. "You shouldn't have done that! Honestly, we can't take you anywhere!"

Jacki, in her quiet way lets me know it was "very rude". I want to tell them that the woman got off lightly with just a little scare after what she put me through. But dammit! I still can't speak well enough to express myself. This will have to wait for another time when I can. For now I'll have to keep the joke to myself. I laugh inside my head all the way down to the Speech Therapy department.

We're greeted at Speech Therapy like old friends. Jaki and Sue chatter away comfortably. I have no idea who Alisa and Brian are. But I'm drowned in suspicion as the smiling Alisa immediately tells me how good I look after my time at rehab.

"Did you send me?" I snap, preparing for battle.

She looks a little uncomfortable. "Actually, no...Brian and I tried very hard to have you sent to a closer rehab where we could continue working with you."

My hackles settle down. I still don't recognize these people until suddenly a flashback hits me. Oh no! The banana and the Christmas

Carol!

I'm not disappointed that Sacramento is taking its sweet time approving my voucher for Speech Therapy. More bananas and Christmas Carols I don't need.

What I do need is money! Jaki and Sue have been advised, however, not to put too much pressure on the state at one time. "Get MediCal squared away before you request disability insurance or it will be a nightmare of confusion," so advise workers at the hospital.

This means I have to exist on my very small monthly annuity of $133.17. It sounds impossible but it's amazing what you can do when you have to. Luckily Jaki set aside a year and a half of rent money from the small funds I had so at least I have a roof over my head.

Megan's Photo Gallery From the 1960's

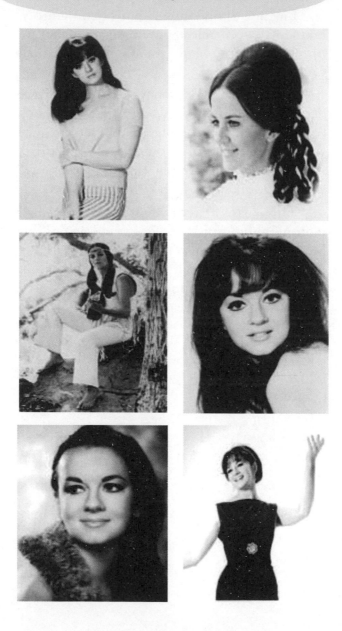

nineteen

Megan Timothy

Another Crisis

"You're rubbing your eyes again. Are you tired?" Jaki asks as we work on my reading.

"Not tired...but...," I blink rapidly, wishing the fuzzy part at the edge of my eyes would disappear. "It's just, well...just...um...I'm not sure whether to blame my brain or my eyes. I know I still have a spelling problem, but I seem to miss seeing the actual letters until you point them out."

Jaki arranges for her friend, Elena Kern's husband, who's an ophthalmologist in Hemet, to check my eyes. Since I'm still not approved by MediCal, the visit is gratis - yet another kindness. People continue to amaze me.

Dr. Kern confirms the fear I've been avoiding. The AVM destroyed a significant amount of my peripheral vision. My right eye is especially bad. The damage is irreparable.

Although this is something I was half expecting, to have it confirmed is devastating. I sit alone in the dark at home fighting to swim the ever-rising tide of losses that seem determined to drown me. I feel I'm going under. And I'm just too worn out to keep swimming anymore.

I'm about as low, emotionally, as I've been since this whole debacle began. Just as I'm sure I'm drowning in a inky-black pool of despair, Coon Cat comes along demanding her nightly grooming and Petromalt treat. She's too old and frail to groom herself anymore and demands that I do it for her. She doesn't put up with any excuses.

Coon Cat - now there's a soul who has made good use of her nine lives, plus a few more I suspect she's negotiated. She's a survivor if ever I've known one. If she can keep going then so can I. Resolve and determination don't come rushing in, but they begin edging my negativism out of the way. I must focus on what I have, not what I have not.

I still have both my eyes. They might not be perfect as eyes go, but they see pretty well straight ahead. They both made it all the way down the eye chart this morning. Sure, I've been walking into things but now that I know what's wrong I can learn to compensate. The same goes for my reading.

Knowledge, as usual, is the key.

The fear and depression brought on by not facing up to my problem begin to dissipate. Coon Cat has once again worked her feline magic.

I'm now able to clearly see that my glass really is half full, not half empty!

twenty

Alisa

I'm not happy. It's been agreed, not by me, but by Jaki, Sue, and Alisa, and approved by MediCal-Pending that I'm to have speech therapy twice a week. I'd rather be shoveling horse poop at the ranch. I fret over the time and distance it takes to get to and from Moreno Valley. I don't know how Jaki and Sue, even alternating the trip, will be able to keep it up.

Instead of a couple of weeks to a month, I'm told to expect the therapy to take up to two years. Two years! How many frigging letters does Alisa think there are in the alphabet?

Sue and Jaki chat away in front of the car while I sit in the back and brood. I resent the very thought of this hopeless therapy stuff. Honestly, I'm getting on just fine by myself. I've almost memorized half of the alphabet and last night I read two sentences of a newspaper article to Jaki. Yes, it did take me nearly forty minutes but I'll be a lot faster once I've gotten the rest of the alphabet down pat.

We all crowd into Alisa's tiny office. My heart drops another fifty feet. She looks about twenty years old. What on earth is she going to be able to teach me? I just hope she doesn't bring up anything about bananas.

Jaki and Sue ask a lot of questions and make notes. I can't keep up with their rapid chatter.

Alisa congratulates both Jaki and Sue for the work they've been doing with me. "During the first days after a brain injury, stimulation is crucial to reactivate the brain," she says. "It's essential that the brain is not allowed further debilitation. If so, it risks its ability to recover sufficiently." This piece of information gets me all riled up again over Ratchett's lethargy and apparent indifference.

Alisa hands me a pencil and asks me to write a few simple words. I can't. Behaving like a sullen five-year-old, I tell her I've learned half the alphabet and will be reading and writing in no time at all.

"I know this is very difficult for you," she says.

"How would you know?" I grumble silently to myself.

Almost as though she reads my mind, she continues, "Four years ago I had a bad car accident that left me with brain damage similar to yours."

I stare at her.

"I know how impatient you are to get your life back together, but it's going to take time and there are no shortcuts." I sit up and push aside my five-year-old pout. Alisa not only has a college education, she has core experience. She has walked in my shoes, felt the pain, swallowed the anguish.

Some things only life experience can teach. The taste of an apricot, for example, can't be explained in words. To know the taste you must experience it. Verbal descriptions do not give the sensory sensation. Thus, learning will convey only part of the meaning. Alisa has both knowledge and experience.

I have found my teacher and it doesn't matter how old she is. I look into her eyes - really look. She knows! I'm with someone who has traveled my path.

Adrenalin pumps through me.

I dust off hopelessness and set out for a new beginning.

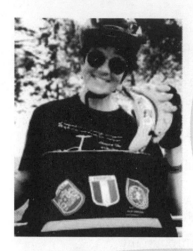

Megan's solo bike ride through Eurpoe, the Middle East, and N. Africa was partially supported by Dole, who provided a steady supply of bananas to keep her fueled.

Megan poses in front of the Salvador Dali museum in Figuero, Spain.

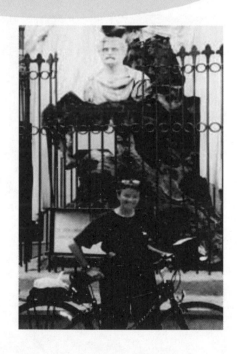

twenty-one

Back On Track

Christmas comes and goes and a New Year slips in. I'm so busy helping at the ranch and working on my reading program with Alisa I hardly notice. My work with Alisa is progressing so well that Jaki no longer has to coach me at night. I'm quite able to manage my homework on my own.

Sue has helped get me back on track with my computer and I've started to e-mail friends - after a fashion. My spelling is still so oddly creative spell-check gives up trying to correct it. My confused friends have invented a dinner party word game featuring my one-of-a-kind e-mails.

Jaki voices her concern when I start walking the six miles to town to do errands. Convinced I'll become lost she puts a large card in my purse with my name, address, and phone number, and her name and phone number and those of all her friends. Just about everyone in the town of Hemet is either listed on my card or alerted to keep an eye out for me. I'm almost too well looked after.

Walking to town is not a casual whim. It's very important to me to spend unhurried time in places like the supermarket. I need to re-familiarize myself with everyday items. Although I've practiced, I still have trouble sorting out the "Fruit on the Bottom" and "Pre-mixed Fruit" yogurt. Making change at the register also flusters me.

While everyone I meet is very kind and helpful, it is not enough. I need to be able to depend on myself and I'll only accomplish that in endless repetition.

The workers at the market are becoming used to me. They no longer regard me with suspicion when I fondle bags of rice and beans muttering to myself and sometimes asking them to pronounce the mysterious letters r-i-c-e and b-e-a-n-s.

The twelve-mile round trip walk, while exhausting, is well worth the effort. My confidence and independence are soaring.

Still, I'm greedy. I want more. I want life in its fullest and to me that means to create.

My books, now lining their shelves, still remain silent. The pieces of wood I've collected to sculpt remain nothing more than old logs. The garden I planned for Jaki is nothing but raw dirt with no vision in mind. There is nothing alive in my head to make the books sing, to create recognizable forms out of the old pieces of wood or a living garden in the pile of desert dirt.

I used to visualize form and color in everything, not only pictorial representations but also words and numbers. Every word I spoke or heard danced with color. My name "Megan" manifests the color rose, the word "good" - yellow, "bad" - black, "flower" - white, "mother" - pink,

"Thursday" – blue. Every letter and number came color coded to my brain.

I was a teenager before I discovered not everyone saw life in color as I did. Because it sounded weird to most people, I kept quiet about it. But I pitied those who lived in a dull colorless world and even dreamed in black and white. It hardly seemed worth the effort to live and dream without color. And now I'm experiencing what a sad life that is.

The few broken words I have are nothing but pale, dirty grey. And sound? Yes, I enjoy the animal sounds but there's no human-created sound in my life. Music, that vital cornerstone of wholeness in a human being is missing.

The Muse, patroness of this magical art form, has taken care to limit the creative gift of making music to a few privileged souls. The rest of us eagerly crave the kaleidoscopic echoes so that we, too, may be graced with its energy.

Music is the stuff that reflects our emotions and enhances the harmony of our spirit. But now silence is my constant companion. I'm afraid to listen to music. I fear sounds that may rattle my injured brain and pummel it with pain.

Or, is it noise and not the sound of music that causes me trouble? Maybe it's time I try discriminating between them and risk a moment of discomfort in order to find the musical solace again.

I brace myself and carefully turn on the radio. Mozart's perfect "Concerto for Clarinet in A" softly floats across the airwaves into my ears and gently caresses my battered brain. There is no assault. Instead, I find healing. I'm comforted and fed the spiritual nourishment I need. There is no suggestion of the audible abuse I feared.

In that moment, I realize now, how emotionally starved I have been. The music calls out to the parts of me derelict and abandoned by the horror of the AVM. And they respond. Not immediately, for they're still afraid, but slowly they start their long journey home.

When I close my eyes now, I see hints of color in my mind. While the books still fail to sing to me, images of form and color for the new gardens are beginning to emerge in my mind. I must get into the dirt and plant!

Something is stirring. I feel it. The music heralds it. Those neglected parts of my head are only asleep, not dead.

I believe this New Year will be a good one!

twenty-two

Fire!

I spoke too soon. My trial is not yet over. Fire is about to purge both me and this land where I live.

When you think of the desert you rarely think of fire. What is there to burn but sand? But here in the deserts of Southern California, wild fires have raged since late summer. Swiftly outgrowing their modest beginnings in mesquite and tumbleweed, they now lust rapaciously for man-made things. The fires explode fire-balls that fly a mile or more ahead of the front, creating a blitzkrieg of a thousand homes and farms. Towers of flame grow so immense they generate their own wind-storm patterns that surge above the mountains and hurtle through the canyons.

The fire has no mercy. It exists only to please its master, the desert winds. Its mission is to deliver on demand the ashes of man and his dwellings, wild beasts, and all other growing things in its path.

Such a fire now threatens the ranch where Jaki and I live. Poised for the fire's potential arrival and the order to evacuate, sleep does not come easily. Dawn delivers an eerie orange glow raining ash from enormous plumes of acrid smoke.

But the fire that invades my house this dawn is not the snarling desert devil. Its smoke is a different color. I can't identify its pungent odor since my sense of smell is yet another part of me that has been damaged by my brain injury.

A smoke alarm screams a warning. Then, another screams and, yet, another. Flames race along beneath the floor under my feet and burst out of the heating ducts. I grab the phone but can't make sense of what I need to do. I only have time to grab Coon Cat and scream for Jaki, next door.

The crisis confronts me with the chilling realization that my brain still does not function well under stress. Faced head-on with an emergency it goes to pieces. I cannot even find, or recognize, the 911 emergency number on the telephone. The truth is, I'm still hopelessly dependent.

The firemen arrive and with cool efficiency have the fire out in an amazingly short time. While all is not lost, the floor of my bathroom and laundry room are gone. Walls, windows, and outside steps are just shells. Water drips. Foam covers everything like icing on a chocolate cake.

The firemen blame a rat or a rabbit for the disaster. There is evidence that something has been chewing on the electrical cables underneath the house.

I'm faint with relief not to be responsible for the blaze. The thought of banishment to "The Place" because of being a threat to myself and others struck me the moment I saw the flames. I cannot admit I lack the simple ability to dial 911. My fear of being sent back to "The Place" is way too strong. I cannot survive living as a "throw away" ever again!

Why is it, that in this wealthy country where we consider ourselves civilized, we are so intolerant and quick to judge? Just because I can't speak the same language as others right now, doesn't give anyone the right to toss me aside as though I'm a piece of garbage.

I will survive this ordeal and be whole again!

And I'll never go back to "The Place" or any of its kin, ever again!

Just a few hours ago Jaki had a guest house and I had a safe haven. Now we share black soot and burnt out walls.

My life has become too absurd to take seriously. I want to laugh. I need to put some emotional distance between me and this latest disaster and laughter's one of the best ways to do that. Jaki and I look at each other wordlessly and start laughing. Laughter turns to tears...then finally back to laughter.

This small drama has already passed beyond the rest of nearby life. Crops are being harvested from the market garden next door. Neighbors walk their dogs. UPS delivers packages. And news arrives that the horrendous wild fires in our area are finally out.

Much later, in the early hours, I sit in my burnt-out bedroom nursing numbed shock. It's that quiet time when the nocturnal animals have gone to rest and their daytime friends have not yet awakened. It's the time when night and day become one. Lovers lie locked in the fierce erotica that drives them to procreate as dawn breaks. Roosters herald the new day's fledgling birth. Our mother, Lady Moon, strains in the agony of delivery. Her child, Sun, bursts into life on the horizon.

I see it as a new birth for myself. And like a newborn child, I stand naked, stripped of most of my earthly possessions. I'm washed clean like the new day. I have been purged but not by demons.

My ravaged brain has emerged with clearer thoughts. The material things I valued were nothing but clutter. They're nothing!

Now, with nothing of value left but my soul, I have found freedom.

As the sun moves higher in the clear, blue sky, I know that true freedom offers peace.

Hollywood

This week my roller coaster life is on an upswing. Lisa, my agent, calls to tell me there's some interest in my screenplay, "In Pursuit of a King". I urge Jaki and Sue not to get overly excited. If ever there's a fickle mistress it's Hollywood. Words rarely mean a thing. Even a check in hand is not good enough. You wait until it's cashed and the money is in your pocket before you celebrate.

Lisa calls again. "The producers want to meet with you next week," she tells me.

I can't help quivering with excitement. I'm being noticed as a real, live, functioning human being. My work has garnered attention. The rush is intoxicating. I revel in it, swallow it, roll around in it, paint myself with it. I have a lot of fun until reality shows up.

Truth is I'm in no condition for any kind of formal meeting, least of all with a room full of Hollywood sharks. They'll eat me alive.

Writers rarely manage to claw their way up to the first rung in Hollywood. And most writers over thirty lie dead in the water.

The thought of the expressions on the producers faces at the sight of me makes me giggle. A sixty-one-year-old-writer? A woman! A sixty-one-year-old-woman-writer with one eye and half a brain!!!

Lisa sees my point and agrees to arrange a conference call in place of the face to face. Being out of sight will definitely be to my advantage.

I really need the money. Even a paltry option would seem like a fortune after existing on $133.17 a month.

Thankfully, I don't have to struggle to re-read the script. Even though I wrote it some years ago and I'm emerging from brain trauma, the story remains fresh in my mind. What concerns me is what I've come to describe as my "constipated words". I know what I feel, what I comprehend, what I wish to express. It's verbalizing these thoughts that continues to trap me. Instead of flowing freely they back up like flood debris in a raging river.

My mind has but a tiny pinhole to free the flood of words trapped in my head, thus constipating the expression of my thoughts.

I spend days planning my strategy for the meeting, not only running the complex non-fictional, historically accurate story over in my mind, but verbalizing the characters and situations.

I'm ready.

The phone rings.

I take a deep breath. Then, suddenly I'm not at all sure I am ready.

Introductions go well. Happy to hear the sound of their own voices, the producers launch into conversation between each other. I'm happy to be ignored - the silent writer. The conversation among the producers intensifies. One of them decides that the minor female character should be re-written as a "hot" love interest.

"But Cecil Rhodes had no interest in women," I remind him.

There's a brief silence.

"So what? Make him straight!" he growls.

"This isn't fiction! Cecil John Rhodes was one of the most powerful men in British Colonial Africa in the late nineteenth century..." I assert.

"What's the name of that woman...the adventuress?" he asks, brushing me off. They're determined to have it their way.

But, I'm desperate for money, so something has to give. History flies out the window. As stress reels in my words I rush to get out the woman's name. But the pinhole clamps shut just as I'm about to spit it out. My eyes hopelessly search my prepared notes.

Too late! The writing dances around making no sense at all.

I'm in meltdown. There's no way I'm able to read. I'm left with only one option and that's a long shot to say the least.

Recently I created a way to retrieve lost words in a roundabout fashion. I doubt these Hollywood producers will have the patience for it since they insist on everything being explained in three words and preferably fewer seconds. But I have no choice. It's all I have and it's vital I deliver this woman's name.

I take a deep breath and launch into my eccentric word-finding process.

"What is the name of the American president assassinated in 1963?"

Silence.

If nothing else, I have their attention.

"Aren't we discussing the late nineteenth century?" one of the producers asks.

"Yes, yes. But bear with me, please."

"Are you talking about Kennedy?"

"Yes! What was his wife's name?"

An even longer silence followed by an uncomfortable cough. "Jacqueline?"

"Yes!" My heart beats fiercely. Can I hang onto these restless Hollywood moguls who are fast losing patience with this bizarre game of charades? "What's the name of Jackie Kennedy's sister...the Princess?"

"Lee Radziwill?"

"That's it! That's it! The nineteenth century adventurer who involved Cecil John Rhodes in an unsavory scandal was the Polish princess, Catherine Radziwill!"

The lads on the other end of the phone don't share my triumph or celebrate my ingenuity. After a brief heavy silence they hang up. But I'm very proud of myself. I managed to untangle the answer without collapsing. I do remember things. I can find answers even if the route to them is somewhat circuitous.

Of course the whole deal goes down the drain and I'm back to my $133.17 a month life style.

But I'm excited. I didn't fold under pressure. I stuck it out and found the answer. I couldn't have done this three months ago.

I may not be ready for prime time, but I'm truly on my way!

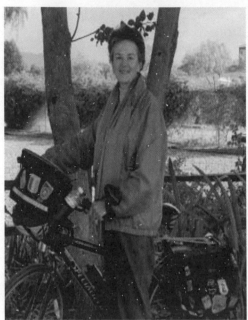

Photo by Jessica Busby

Megan thinks nothing
of riding her bike 7 or 8 miles into Hemet
to shop for food or attend her reading
class at the Library.

twenty-four

Triumphs and Challenges

I may not have wowed Hollywood yesterday, but today, in the dairy section of supermarket, I redeemed myself. Following an exceptionally garrulous bout of threats and strong language, the recalcitrant yogurt tubs finally capitulate. The words on their labels explode like popcorn in a hot pot - "Fruit on the Bottom"! "Pre-mixed Fruit"! The muddled letters form real words! I roll them around on my tongue, toy with them, toss them back and forth. I no longer have to pursue them hither and yon.

Instead, the mercurial poltergeists come to heel, tamed. They flow unswervingly from mind to lip holding form, balanced and steadfast.

"Fruit on the Bottom, Fruit on the Bottom, Fruit on the Bottom, FRUIT... ON... THE... BOTTOM!" I sing out to startled shoppers. Who says a sonnet needs fourteen words when just four create perfection?

Soon after my success with the yogurt, my cycling friends, Nancy and Richard Wedeen come down from L.A. to visit. Richard works on my bike all day and leaves me with wheels! It's wonderful to get to town in less than half an hour compared to the hour and a half it's been taking me to walk. The measured pace of a bicycle gives me confidence and time for my damaged eyes to take into consideration the perils of the road. My bike's panniers offer the option of carrying up to forty pounds, more than enough for any shopping I need to do including heavy items such as three one-gallon bottles of water. It gives me a real feeling of independence. I no longer have to ask for any help getting around town. Jaki and Sue, however, continue to cart me back and forth to Moreno Valley for my bi-weekly sessions with Alisa.

I thought that after mastering the alphabet and my success with "Fruit on the Bottom" everything else involving speaking, reading, and writing would just fall into place. I'm wrong!

I arrive for my session with Alisa pretty cocky. After a month, except for "g", "u" and a few muddles with "x" and "z", which you hardly ever use anyway, I've got the alphabet under control. "OK, bring on the books...lets read!"

Alisa gently warns me I have a lot more to learn before I can tackle books.

"What do you mean? The alphabet is the alphabet," I argue.

"Shut up and listen!" Sue mutters.

Alisa goes on to talk a lot about "building blocks".

"Building blocks? I have no ambition to be a structural engineer. I just want to read!"

"Then you'd better listen...LISTEN!" hisses Sue.

I'm not in the mood to be opposed. I've been denied too long and refuse to wait any more. Don't they understand what it is to live in this half world - refused knowledge and information? Alisa should know! She's been to this dark side of life. Why does she, of all people, deny me?

I continue to be a querulous kvetch. Sue is close to whacking me on my shins.

Alisa remains quiet and calm waiting for me to exhaust myself. Then she quietly explains that mastering the alphabet is not just learning to recognize its letters visually but to learn their sounds.

"Of course I know the sounds," I fume.

She writes something down and turns it around to me. "What does this say?" She's written A - B - C.

"A,B,C!" I recite sarcastically rolling my eyes.

"Yes, but what do they SAY...what are their SOUNDS?"

I stare at the letters I've used for sixty-one years and I haven't a clue. Sue looks at me, her face expressionless except for a slightly raised eyebrow which says more than a thousand words.

"Okay, okay! I admit I'm a jerk. I apologize. It's just that I want this so badly."

"I know," says Alisa, "and you will have it! But remember your reading is starting from scratch...and I mean SCRATCH! There are no short cuts...this is a very difficult road but I know you have the strength to make it."

I stop wasting time and misjudging those on

my side and start learning zealously. I'm amazed to find many letters have more than one sound. "A" has the nerve to come up with four!

"A" for ape -

"A" for apple -

"A" for awful —

and "A" for Alisa.

I learn all the letter sounds only to find Alisa has more tricks up her sleeve. There are vowels which have their own complicated sounds - not to mention consonants that fly off in all directions. "Ph" insists on sounding like an "f" most of the time. "Igh" totally ignores the "gh" part so why on earth has someone bothered to put it in? And what about "tion", "sion", "cion" all making a "shun" sound? Now where the heck does that come from?

Alisa is not done with me yet but she does help by drawing little pictures on the cards she's made for me. A cute mouse stealing cheese to remind me that "ch" says "ch" as in cheese. A shoe for "sh", a mitten indicates a thumb for "th". Alisa makes me stacks of cards that take me months to learn.

How did I ever learn all this so easily as a child? How do kids today manage? One thing I do know is that the person who created the English language deserves to be hung, drawn, and quartered - even if he'd have to be dug up to do it!

I realize I have to learn how to maneuver a

brain whose parts run at different speeds. Some parts cruise along at eighty miles an hour and others, like my reading function, labor at just about one mile an hour, if that. This is something I believe I'm going to have to work out for myself. No one can see inside my head. Each brain creates its own complexities, detailing its fine tuning to its personal whim. My brain sometimes even surprises the experienced and brilliant Alisa - for instance, with its comprehension and retention.

People with brain damage such as mine may learn to read, but their comprehension and memory are often weak or practically non-existent. Not only do I understand what I read, but, if Alisa asks me about a certain passage a week later, I can relate it in detail, not verbatim, but using my own words, as primitive as they are. If she gives me a familiar sentence to read I remind her I already read it two weeks ago.

Yet my words remain constipated and it is still very difficult to express myself and find needed words without performing the whole rigmarole that freaked out the movie moguls.

But while the whole thing continues to be very much a mystery, things are starting to drop into place. My work with Alisa continues to go well even if I do argue a lot. My argumentative nature has become a joke among us. I start off each session with an apology just to make sure I've got good credit in the bank - because I know that as sure as the sun rises and sets I will have spent it before the hour is over.

Let Me Die Laughing!

twenty-five

Books, Glorious Books!

I have to read a book. I absolutely have to! Yes, I understand the building blocks are my road to achieving my goal. But the unrelenting practice, practice, practice - the same every day, all day, with no end to the repetition - threatens to grind down my soul. Vowel sounds, sight words, practice words, phonic rules, double consonants, etc, etc, etc, etc!!!

Did I ever carry so many details in my brain? And will I ever cement all these slippery little devils back? A couple good sentences with the Hollywood moguls and conquering "Fruit on the Bottom" and I screech to a halt. I must read a book!

Sitting alone, day after day, practicing the alphabet sometimes drives me close to madness. Fancy reciting the ABC's when you're sixty-one years old! I have to read a book.

I have to read a book!

I don't care if Alisa, Jaki, Sue or anyone else tells me I'm not ready, that attempting to read a book at this stage will only frustrate me. I'm going to do A BOOK!

I stare at my book shelves feeling as if I'm about to raid a candy store. My mouth waters for one of the forbidden bonbons. I reach for a young adult book, _Young Joan_ - a remarkable novel on the childhood of Joan of Arc. Not only is the courageous Joan of Arc an inspiration but so is the author, Barbara Dana. A woman of grace and courage herself, she gave me this book some years ago. I feel both Barbara's spirit and Joan of Arc's are with me.

I start.

"Our house is made of stone with a slanted roof..."

It's very difficult. After the first paragraph, only three sentences, I'm exhausted. It has taken me half an hour but I'm exhilarated. The words made sense which means I got them right.

Tonight I started to read a book!

I stay awake long after I turn out the light. It's wonderfully exciting to have taken the first steps of this journey I long for so much.

I take the book to class, eager to surprise Alisa. But I'm too eager, too excited. I thrash around like a caged monkey desperate to get through a short paragraph, or just one sentence. Please!

I don't dare stop trying – dare not raise my eyes to Alisa.

I have to succeed!

Minutes tick by as sweat pours down my face.

I will not fail!

I will not!

But...

I do.

Devastated, I keep my eyes down.

This is exactly what Alisa said would happen. But instead of reproof, having walked this road herself, she understands. "While I'm obviously not going to be able to persuade you not to read at this point, I do think we should try to figure out a different approach." Her support prompts my failing hopes to bounce back. "You might," she adds, "experiment with combining both visual and audio of the same book."

I don't have an audio tape for _Young Joan_, but Sue has the first _Harry Potter_ book and its accompanying audio tape. Jaki gives me a radio with a tape deck. I start out playing a sentence, repeating it verbally then verbalizing it again both reading the book and listening to the tape. It's laborious.

In the beginning I have to repeat the same sentence again and again. But after a few days I get the rhythm of reading and listening and maintaining my comprehension through the boredom of the repetition.

It's going to work. I feel it in my bones. The tape helps me work out words I don't recognize visually and corrects my verbal errors. After a couple of weeks I begin to use the tape only for corrections. A little later I cut it down to checking paragraphs. After a month I eliminate the tape altogether.

The system's working for me!

I move on to _Harry Potter II_. Because I'm

familiar with the characters and the story-line, it isn't difficult. This doesn't mean to say I'm a speed-reader. I still read at the pace of a young child.

The downside of the relative ease afforded by using the tapes is that it's less of a workout for my brain - a stroll in the park instead of a hike up a steep mountain. I keep up the hiking part by reading short newspaper articles intermittently throughout the day.

I have to control my overwhelming impulse to read by taking a break every half-hour. Alisa insists on this and, of course, she's right. After that length of time the words start to collapse and nothing but rest restores them. A half-hour of reading, especially at my pace, is frustrating but that's the way it is right now. I have to learn to live with it until my brain strengthens.

I balk at _Harry Potter III_. I want to read a "grownup book" and my friend, Jean, has given me _The Da Vinci Code_. My weekly write-up surprises them all. Sue suggests to Alisa that she limit my book reports. "If you don't limit her to half a page we'll all have to work out her spelling in another nine pages next week!"

"Cowards!" I'm intensely excited over my nine pages despite their joshing but do agree to the limit. I continue with _The Da Vinci Code_. It takes me three months to finish it. But I do it. And, more important, I enjoyed it!

My next challenge is to write. Not book

reports, newspaper reviews, or e-mails, but to really write. There's no more room to store words in my head. They have to come out to the light of day and get down on paper.

Let Me Die Laughing!

twenty-six

Anniversary

It's the first anniversary of my Big Bang and my gift is a MediCal card. The real thing! I no longer have to skulk around with the rest of the MediCal-Pending orphans. I've been adopted. I'm one of the family.

My gift qualifies me for an MRI (magnetic-resonator-imaging), an expensive procedure to check the condition of my brain. I had an MRI the day of my "incident", so I'm told. But my memory during those twilight days is fuzzy at best and the MRI totally failed to register.

I realize the value of that oblivion the moment I'm thrust into the MRI machine, a trash compactor-like bin with barely space to breathe. My highly-claustrophobic senses take off like a space rocket. Horrendous crashing noises, reminiscent of a 6.8 California earthquake, send my super-sensitive ears somewhere into outer space. I'm too stunned to move, think, or even panic. I just lie stupefied. An hour and a half later I'm dragged out dripping with sweat and astonished to find not only myself, but the rest of California still in one piece.

We arrive at Dr. K's office to hear the results of the MRI. Whatever it takes I know I must get off the medication. I'm now on my fourth variety of anti-seizure drugs and have paid for each with one nasty side effect or another. The first turned me into a boiled lobster. The second made my hair fall out of my head and grow on my chin. Next I'm either driven to constipation or diarrhea. The latest, Neurontin, leaves me constantly tired and fighting depression.

I've given so much blood for the frequent tests required to keep track of the effects, it's a wonder I have any left. All the tests show my liver and kidneys are under stress. Where will it end if I have to keep compensating for side effect after side effect?

I see many patients in the hospital leaving the pharmacy with a supermarket bag full of drugs. It scares me half to death. One man showed me his stash of sixteen bottles. He admits sorting, timing, and medicating himself is a 24/7 job. I have no interest in that kind of life.

The noise and the crowds at Moreno Valley Hospital are almost too much for my sensitive brain to tolerate. Alarms ring, hospital pagers squawk, people chatter raucously on their cell phones. We're perpetually reminded we're in a state institution. Armed guards constantly escort prisoner/patients clad in bright orange jump-suits and rattling shackles chained to their waists.

Civilian patients along with their families and friends strive to ward off boredom waiting hours to see a doctor. Besides the usual games of checkers and mind-numbing TV, beauty preparation is a popular pastime. We're entertained by eyebrow pluckers, and makeup artists, cornrow braiding, short hair cuts, manicures, pedicures and nail art. Parents don't seem at all concerned that their children shoot popcorn at anything or anyone. Some families, making themselves comfortable on the floor, set up picnic lunches. Half the time you swear you're at Disneyland not a hospital.

The Neurology Department appears to be more sober minded - no picnics or beauty preparations allowed in there. Dr. K scans my MRI pictures clipped to the light board. "Well," she says, "it looks as if you're ready to proceed with treatment. You have three choices. One, you can do nothing. At present you have a four-percent chance of having another incident, which will increase at the rate of four percent per annum. You will, of course, have to continue with the anti-seizure medication."

"For how long?" asks Jaki.

"For the rest of her life."

The first part sounds like a pretty acceptable risk considering I'm sixty-one but the second is totally unacceptable. The side-effects of the powerful anti-seizure drugs are not something I'm prepared to live with. There's a good possibility they could add other health problems which would have to be counteracted by more drugs. I can't see the point of solving one problem while knowingly creating others.

"The second option," Dr. K continues, "is to have radiation therapy...a painless outpatient procedure."

This is getting worse! I'm not enamored over having my brain involved with radiation. The word itself scares me out of my wits.

"Your third option is to have brain surgery...however..." she hesitates, reviewing the MRI pictures again, "I'm not sure your condition can tolerate surgery."

I'm appalled by the menu of options offered by Dr. K. "Do nothing", "fry what's left of my brain", or "slice and dice". Where's my silver bullet?

I'm running on empty, dazed and confused. To be able to make any kind of decision as to how to regain some semblance of control in my life, I need more information. I need clear understanding of my condition, not just the vague answers that have been offered to me up to now. I must gain true understanding of what has happened and what directions are open to me.

I need to do research. But to do that I have to have the ability to read at a much higher level than what I currently am able. Tough luck! I feel isolated. Everyone around me speaks too fast and uses words I don't understand.

Later, when I'm alone with Jaki and Sue I feel better. It's quiet in the house. I can breathe again and ask questions with answers patiently explained to me. After some discussion we all come to agreement that the lesser of the three evils appears to be radiology treatment.

Since there is no appropriate radiation facility at Moreno Valley we're sent even further afield to Loma Linda University Medical Center. There Jaki and I meet with the Radiation Medicine Physician, Dr. Maria Simental, who studies my MRI, then confirms radiation therapy could well be the answer but...

"The success of the procedure will not be known for three years..."

"What do you mean, three years?" I ask with a sinking feeling in the pit of my stomach.

"It takes three years before we can be assured of its success."

"And what do I do in the meantime?" I ask, working hard not to scream.

"You will stay on the medication..."

My words now topple into a muddle as they always do when I'm stressed, so Jaki takes over. "Can you guarantee success?"

"Her chances appear good but there are never any guaranties."

"What are her options should the procedure not succeed?"

"Surgery." That word again.

I'm devastated. Dr. Simental, seeing our disappointment, tries to make amends "Here's a name," she says scribbling on a piece of paper. "I highly recommend this surgeon...he's a brilliant man. However, he's extremely busy and difficult to get in touch with."

We're half-way out the door when she calls, "Wait! It's a long shot but let me call Dr. Hsu's office." She returns minutes later with a big smile. "You have no idea how lucky you are. He can see you in fifteen minutes!"

As Jaki hurries me along she warns that brilliant brain surgeons are notorious for their egos. I really couldn't care less. No stranger, monstrous ego or otherwise, is going to dig around in my head. I'm only going along for the ride because Jaki's so eager.

Having been warned of Dr. Hsu's busy schedule we don't expect more than a brief visit. Instead we're received cordially as if time were no object. It's clear that ego and attitude are not Dr. Hsu's style. Like many truly brilliant people he doesn't need them. He displays his intelligence with the effortless grace of someone who has found peace and comfort within himself. It's both impressive and comforting to be in the company of such a man. His calm demeanor immediately gives me a sense of security.

"*Wait a minute!*" my analytical side shouts. "*Don't give me 'impressive'…he's a surgeon…give him a minute and he'll be into your head with a scalpel!*" As I watch Dr. Hsu carefully scan my MRI pictures, I'm trying desperately to reconcile my internal conflict. My instinct tells me to trust him, but my logical side yells "*Slow down! Slow down! You may be impressed by this man but remember he's a neurosurgeon about to offer you a potentially life-threatening procedure. Just a few minutes ago you vowed you'd never ever think of having brain surgery. What's wrong with you?"*

There's no time to continue the argument with myself. Dr. Hsu turns to face us. "You have a very serious situation but I do believe I can help you."

"See! You have a serious problem," my analytical side bellows.

"Shut up and listen!" my intuition shouts back.

Sensitive to the fright in my eyes, Dr. Hsu invites both Jaki and me to step up to the MRI pictures. There, all angles of my brain are displayed in dozens of tiny pictures. Dr. Hsu begins to explain my situation and for the first time, either because I'm finally ready to face my position head-on or because I've found someone I really trust, I allow my mind to open and I hear and understand most of what he's saying. Here in this quiet room, listening to this gentle man's quiet, unhurried voice, I finally begin to get a handle on where I stand.

"An Arterio-Venous-Malformation, or AVM," says Dr. Hsu, "is a rare condition affecting about 250,000 people in the United States. It's an abnormal collection of blood vessels which can be thought of as a 'short circuit'. The blood, instead of nourishing the tissues in the brain, pumps straight back to the heart without ever giving nutrients to the tissues."

"What causes it?" I ask.

"It's a congenital defect caused by a rupture or clotting during fetal development before birth."

Although I'd already been told having an AVM is not my fault it's good to hear it again from Dr. Hsu. "The danger of this abnormality is that patients are seldom aware they have it until they suffer a bleed..."

"Not an explosion?" I ask.

"No, a bleed," Dr. Hsu repeats with a faint smile.

"Megan always opts for the dramatic," Jaki says, ruefully.

Dr. Hsu smiles again. "You have three options," continues Dr. Hsu running through the same list given to us by Dr. K. He sketches a chart itemizing a list of the advantages and disadvantages of the options. "Doing nothing" starts off as the safest but increases its danger over time. Radiation is also a good bet to start with but then where does it go? It offers no answers for three long, scary years. Surgery delivers its danger right up front and that's a serious one, obviously. But pass that hurdle and you're home free. I appreciate Dr. Hsu's candor. His simple explanation definitely helps clarify my options.

With all the cards on the table I can set about making a decision. And it will be MY decision. Having gained some control of my life, I feel better than I have since the start of this debacle. Better, until a big "but..." rings out from

Dr. Hsu. Here we go...the invariable "but". My heart sinks remembering Dr. K's warning that there might be a problem with surgery. Has my optimism made me jump the gun again? I brace myself.

Dr. Hsu draws a quick sketch. "This might be a problem." He taps his pen on something that looks like the tail feather of a molting chicken. "If the AVM, starting here, at the end of the posterior cerebral artery, goes too deep into this...it's called Labbe's Vein, or the Labbe'...surgery will be too dangerous. I can't tell from these pictures exactly where the Labbe' goes.

"And what procedure will clarify that?" asks Jaki.

"An outpatient procedure called an angiogram. We would insert dye into Megan's brain to give us the information we need regarding the exact route of the Labbe'."

A bit later, as we drive away from the clinic my mind is made up. If the angiogram is positive I want Dr. Hsu to be my ally - the one to guide me through this very difficult part of my life. My instinct on this issue is so strong my analytical side can't get a word in edgewise. I feel very calm about it. Despite my initial ambiguity I know I'm doing the right thing. I tell Jaki I'm going to have the surgery if possible.

She's silent for a minute before she answers. "I'd do exactly the same thing if I were in your shoes. I feel really good about Dr. Hsu. There's no way I'd want to live with the risk of another AVM hanging over my head."

When I get home I call Sue with the news. There's a long silence on the phone before she replies. "That's a pretty radical turn-around for you."

"I know it sounds radical but today...for the first time...I really started to think for myself again and I'm convinced I've made the right choice."

Silence.

"Sue? Are you still there?"

"I'm here." Her voice was barely audible.

"I thought you'd be pleased to know I've finally gained enough confidence to strike out on my own."

"Yeah, but, you're supposed to start with baby steps not big jumps...and this is a massive leap!"

"It's never been my style to start small," I insist with a laugh.

"But are you sure..."

"Yes!"

"But you were so adamantly against the very idea of surgery."

"Dr. Hsu changed that. I really feel he's the right person to help me through this ordeal."

"It's a very aggressive course of action to dive into with someone you've only known for half an hour!"

"You'll understand when you meet him."

"He must be a damned good salesman to talk you into it...and that's what he is, you know...a salesman!"

"Come and meet him when I see him after the angiogram."

"Oh, I can't wait! Megan, Megan, are you really sure..."

"Yes! Yes, I am. If it gives you any comfort, I have to pass the angiogram test before I get the okay for surgery and I can cancel at any time if I change my mind."

"Small comfort is better than none I suppose...but..."

"My instinct tells me..."

"You're going on your instinct? Oh, Megan!"

"It's never failed me before, Sue."

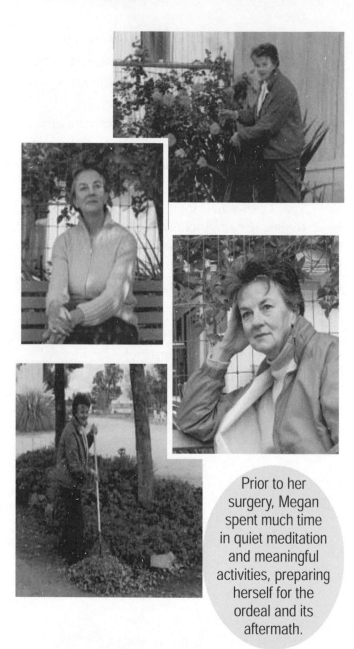

Prior to her surgery, Megan spent much time in quiet meditation and meaningful activities, preparing herself for the ordeal and its aftermath.

Photos by Jessica Busby

Dr. Hsu

I emerge from the angiogram with the good news that the questionable Labbe' near the AVM will not hamper my plans for surgery. Both Jaki and Sue join me for a conference with Dr. Hsu - Jaki supportive, Sue dubious. Sue makes sure I remember that my decision to have the surgery is not carved in stone and that the option to change my mind still exists. I've written out a careful list of questions I want to ask Dr. Hsu and have made copies for everyone since I still don't trust myself when it comes to speaking under pressure.

Dr. Hsu arrives accompanied by a psychiatrist who doesn't say much but watches me intently. Dr. Hsu is the same kind, compassionate man I remember meeting two weeks ago. He reviews the information he gave previously, then states clearly, "You are aware that this operation is not a cure."

I nod my understanding.

"It will stop the danger of having another bleed but you will be left with all the damage created by the AVM. Your speaking, reading, and writing abilities will only improve with further intense therapy and hard work on your part."

I nod my understanding again.

His eyes and voice suddenly become expressionless and he appears uncomfortable. "In general the risk level of this surgery ranges from one, the least, to five the most serious. Your risk lies in the three to four range. It's a very difficult and serious operation...and you could die." Both he and the psychiatrist watch me intently.

"Are you testing me?"

Dr. Hsu gives a faint nod. "You might die if you have this operation," he repeats. It appears painfully difficult for him to say this but I suspect it's necessary due to all the malpractice suits flying around.

"Doctor, I'm very aware people die from all sorts of surgical complications. I've heard of someone going in to have their...um...gall bladder out and...well, anyway..." I glanced at Jaki, then at Sue, drew in a breath and said, "It's not death that bothers me. If you're dead you're dead. What concerns me is coming back half baked." Now it's my turn to watch him.

Both men remain silent and expressionless, waiting for me to continue.

"I need your word, Dr. Hsu, that should the surgery not work out as we all hope, I will not be tossed aside into some hell-hole like I was before. That's not just a frightening thought, it's a terrifying one. If I lose everything I've worked to restore over this past year it will be a pity, a great pity, but not the end - not if I'm given the chance to start over. Whatever appears lost when you look at me from the outside, remember somewhere within I have a spirit. It's a powerful one and I need your word that I will be given the opportunity to fight my way back again." This is the longest speech I've given since my AVM and, exhausted, my words fade away.

Dr. Hsu's kind expression returns as does the softness of his voice. "You have my word you will not be tossed aside...and you must believe that I would not do this operation if I thought I wasn't confident I could help you."

Our eyes lock, exchanging truth and trust. No more words are necessary between us.

Sue and Jaki, recognizing I'm done talking for the day, take over asking my list of questions. I learn that not one, but two operations are required. In the first, an embolization, a device is inserted through an opening in the femoral artery and guided to the brain where it will plug some of the blood vessels of the AVM. It will take four or five hours.

The actual AVM surgery will take place early the next morning after another MRI. The AVM surgery is estimated to take six to ten hours. I should be in the hospital for about six days and then in rehabilitation for two weeks.

My mind wanders. I could be away from home for three weeks! I begin to fret about little Coon Cat. She's so frail and requires hydration once, sometimes twice a week. These sessions run about twenty minutes and I know Jaki, who in addition to all the ranch work, has her ailing husband and aging mother to care for. She doesn't have the time for Coon Cat's special needs.

I snap back to the present. Everyone is getting to their feet and Dr. Hsu is urging me to call him if I have any more questions. His last words to me are that the decision whether or not to have the operation is mine and that I'm free to cancel the surgery at any time should I choose.

On the way home Sue admits to coming around to feeling the same about Dr. Hsu as Jaki and I, but she still remains apprehensive about the surgery, itself. I tell her if she comes up with anything better I'd be glad to consider it, but in the meantime she should stop watching PBS medical documentaries.

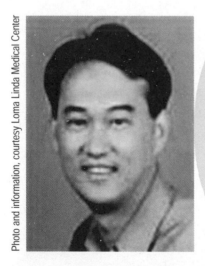

Photo and information, courtesy Loma Linda Medical Center

Dr. Frank P.K. Hsu

Dr. Hsu has special research interests in the biomechanics of cerebral aneurysms, brain and spinal cavernous malformations, and the application of technology within neurosurgery.

twenty-eight

Chasing Money

Prior to going in for brain surgery, I have a list of things I must do. Right at the top of that list is dealing with Social Security. The year-long bureaucratic MediCal nightmare has worn Jaki to the bone. Sue courageously steps up to the plate to shoulder my battle to get Disability Insurance. With nearly two months before my surgery we figure we have ample time to take care of business. We arrive for our appointment at the Social Security Office.

Sue staggers under pounds of medical records that cover the entire history of my AVM. I bring a wad of identification papers - driver's license, passport, old immigration papers and citizenship paper. It's not enough, however, and we're sent out to gather more.

We return a week later. "Who are you? What do you want?" demand the gate-keepers of the Social Security Office. It seems the papers we'd brought on our first visit as well as the new batch we'd filed have completely disappeared. There's doubt whether we were ever here at all.

We start again!

Round two.

We face the same who-are-you, no-such-papers-exist excuse, but this time Sue's prepared. She's arrived with two copies of all the documents and insists on a signed, dated receipt. It causes a flurry and some surly comments but she sticks to her guns.

We are granted an interview...in two weeks. It's questionable if two months will be enough time after all.

D-Day!

We arrive. Mr. S, while pleasant enough, is downright suspicions about my request for disability. There's nothing eye-catching about my brain damage. It's the showy, mangled body parts that get all the attention. True, I can barely speak, read, or write but then that's not unusual, especially with people of suspicious accent such as Sue's and my own. The country's flooded with illegals looking for a hand-out.

Mr. S regards my battered passport with suspicion as he thumbs through its exotic stamps from countries that still retain the old fashion habit of stamping passports. Finally, forced to admit the passport is valid he starts thumbing through Sue's stack of papers.

"What's this?!" he crows holding a bank statement aloft.

"An irrevocable annuity," says Sue.

"Then she does have money!"

"Uh, yeah, one-hundred, thirty-three dollars and seventeen cents a month."

"What's to stop her cashing it? It comes to a few thousand dollars."

"Irrevocable", says Sue, struggling not to

sound sarcastic, "means it cannot be revoked for ANY reason."

"Mm, we'll have to have our legal staff look into it."

It takes a few more visits over a few more weeks before the Social Security Legal Department finally agrees that, indeed, all I can get out of my annuity is $133.17 a month.

And, so we're moved on to be interviewed by Ms. X. I give a lot of thought as to how I should dress for the occasion. Proud of my effort I parade around in front of Sue. "If it's at all possible, do I look poorer than I actually am?"

"I don't know about poor, but it looks as if you slept in your clothes."

"Well, of course I did…it's important I capture that 'homeless-patina' look." I laugh at the thought but realize how close to reality that concept is. Sue offers no praise for ingenuity, only rolls her eyes.

We're summoned to a woman we instantly name the Wicked Witch. We know we're in trouble when she greets us brandishing the notorious irrevocable annuity. "It's a crime to hide money when applying for government assistance," she snarls.

"What?" Sue and I chorus.

"This annuity," she drops it as if it's contaminated, "was established at the time of your alleged illness…"

"It's legally…"

"In September of 2003, the state passed a law that makes moving and hiding monies in such a fashion fraud!"

The upside of this calamity is that neither Sue nor I land in the clink on fraud charges. The downside is that my penalty for not keeping up with the obscure law, which not even the attorney who had suggested the annuity had been aware of, is a four-month freeze on applying for disability insurance.

We were wrong!

Two months is not enough time to sort out Social Security!

twenty-nine

Waiting

Next on my "to-do before surgery" list is preparing myself for extremes of coming home or not coming home. The worst part for me is sorting out and tidying up my belongings. Housekeeping ranks somewhere below zero in my list of fun things to do. Fortunately, I don't have to write a will since I don't have anything to leave anyone.

What's really important is my "Advance Health Care Directive". I have a dozen copies made - one each for Jaki and Sue and lots to hand out at the hospital. I want to be sure no one tries any heroics that'll leave me breathing on a respirator for years on end. I pack the freezer with homemade soups and bread anticipating that I won't be inclined to cook when I get home.

With all my busy-work done, the only thing left is to wait. And for me it is the most difficult part. Once I make up my mind to do something I'm eager to get on with it.

I see tension in my friends' eyes. I hear fear in their voices. Some can't help busting into tears. There are those who can only manage hurried phone calls. Others waste my time and try my patience pleading with me to reconsider my decision. Some are simply too afraid to talk to someone they fear has the audacity to challenge fate. While it's not for me to judge another person's attitude when facing the risk of death, being made to feel like a "dead man walking" is not doing me any good. I have no room for anyone's tears and less for their fear. I need all my strength for myself right now.

I need quiet time - time alone.

I stop answering the phone and speak only to Sue and Jaki.

I've made the decision to have the surgery, but the details of it are in Dr. Hsu's hands. I wouldn't have agreed to the operation if my instinct had registered hesitation. My job now is to prepare myself physically and mentally for the intense ordeal ahead. I need to prepare as if entering a marathon.

I increase my daily hikes and soon have the ability to walk a mile while doing the special breathing exercise Dr. Hsu's nurse taught me. It involves blowing out air rather like a "snorting horse". It's by no means elegant, but I'm assured it will be most helpful in flushing the anesthesia drugs from my lungs following the surgery. Since I'm having two operations within a day of each other, I'm bound to be pretty clogged up with whatever they use.

Besides hiking and working hard around the ranch and in the garden, I also increase yoga to stretch and balance my body and self-hypnosis, which some call meditation, to relax my mind. Calmness settles in, sleep comes easily, and I enjoy feeling fit and healthy.

Time has caught up with me and tomorrow the "Big Show", as I've come to call the surgery, begins. Dr. Hsu is the director, and of course I've cast myself as the "star". Well, why not? It's my show!

Today I need to think calmly and clearly, so I take an extra long walk. The knowledge that I might possibly lose my life tomorrow makes living today powerfully sweet. Its intensity triggers the same kind of rush that used to grip me when jumping a horse over an exceptionally demanding hurdle or pushing to a win at the finish line of a race.

My brain is intensely alive with every touch, feel, sight, and sound. All this draws me especially close to the land. I take off my shoes and feel things I never felt before through the bottoms of my feet. My hands thrill to the touch of grass, rocks, and feathers left by passing birds. I need to absorb this land down deep inside. And even though I no longer have the ability to smell it, today the aroma of the desert runs over and through me. I bury it deep inside myself so I will never forget the glorious gift of its perfume.

Late in the afternoon, cumulus clouds boil over the mountains then flatten across the valley like a collapsed souffle'. The afternoon breeze magically brushes away the low clinging clouds to bid farewell to the sun and welcome the moon. It's that magical 15th night cycle of the lunar month - that very special time when the moon rises in the east at exactly the same time the sun sets in the west. And there, for a brief moment, they embrace the equality of mirror images. This evening I'm privileged to be held between them and for a few precious minutes I experience perfection.

Life has never felt so dazzlingly real to me. I no longer question who or what I am. Ego ceases to exist. I become part of the consciousness of all beings, embraced by the beginning awareness of "nirvana" and the realization that life's greatest gift to us all is laughter.

Although this could be my last night here, instead of fear and sadness, I'm filled with life and the joy of it. I drink it, careful not to spill a drop. A coyote, usually shy creatures, stops and watches me. Is it wishing me well for my big adventure tomorrow? Is it congratulating me for opening my mind to see and feel things I have ignored so long? It dips its head in silent farewell and gracefully trots away.

I arrive home tired, but it's a good, healthy tiredness. I fall asleep easily, listening to an unexpected rain shower washing the desert clean. I'm ready for whatever comes tomorrow, Thursday the 4th of November, 2004.

thirty

The Big Show

Rain has arrived early in the desert this year. Last night an unexpected shower left the morning clouds arguing over whether or not to continue with more rain. I barely finish attending to Coon Cat's hydration when Sue arrives to drive me to Loma Linda. As we start to drive out, Jaki runs out to wish me well.

Passing through the gate, Sue glances at me quizzically. "Are you OK?"

I give her a thumbs up.

"Are you sure? You look so calm... and...heaven knows why... you seem cheerful."

"A month from now I'll probably have the shakes."

"What do you mean, 'a month from now'?"

"That's when I'll probably be having post-crisis hysteria...no time for it now. I need to be alert while I'm in the thick of things."

"I don't think I'll ever understand you. If it were me, I'd be...well, I'd be..."

"We all have our own way of coping," I answer. I can't admit how close I am to asking her to turn around and take me home. Last night while walking in the hills, I thought I had everything under control. Now I'm not so sure I'm ready to venture off to explore the very edge of life as I know it.

But, questions and answers are not the point when it comes to life - experience is. And it's experience that lies ahead. I must keep looking ahead, not backwards. I have to continue striding forward, not begin backpedaling now. Definitely, not now!

The Loma Linda parking lot is packed and we end up having to walk two and a half blocks to the hospital. Sue gives me a hard time the whole way. "What on earth do you have in this bag?" she demands.

"Books."

"Books! It feels as if you've absconded with the entire Hemet Public Library."

I try to take the bag from her. She snatches it away from my grasp. "Not on my watch! You know you're not supposed to pick up anything heavy, and since I've brought you this far I'm determined to deliver you in one piece. I'd just like to know what books have to do with brain surgery?"

"Everything! In the event that things don't go as planned I want to be ready to start over, thus the alphabet book. If everything's okay I'll need my dictionary, thesaurus, the poems of Rumi for my soul, _The No. 1 Ladies' Detective Agency_ for laughs, something by Stephen King for thrills..."

"Okay, okay!" she moans staggering along the wet sidewalk.

After a few moments I quietly admit the

books are my security blanket. Sue stares at me her eyes welling just a bit, "I'm relieved to find you're human after all. I think this is the first time I've ever heard you admit to a need."

Later, as I'm about to be rolled away for the embolization, Sue whispers, "Are you sure? We can stop it right now if you want."

"I'm going through with it," I reply adamantly.

"Okay, I'll see you Tuesday!"

Sue, Jaki, and I have all agreed that phone calls to Dr. Hsu will be enough for the next few days. It doesn't make sense for them to drive for hours just to sit around staring at a comatose body. By Tuesday, we're told, I'll be ready to receive company in a civilized fashion.

The gurney rolls into the surgery. I feel quite at home. The same staff who helped me through the angiogram are here. We're cracking jokes about the "advance directive" I've stuck on my forehead when Dr. Lyh, the physician in charge appears.

He's a brilliant but very serious man who neither appreciates nor approves of us clowning around. Being a bit on edge to begin with, I can't stop laughing. Dr. Lyh removes the offending "advance directive" stuck on my forehead and takes a deep breath. "Ms. Timothy," he scolds, "you are about to embark on a very, very serious operation. You could die!"

I manage to bring my laughter down to a

giggle. "So I'm told," I reply, not having total success looking serious. "But if I die, I hope you'll let me die laughing!"

He stares at me not sure if I'm insane or on drugs. I fade into anesthetic oblivion still laughing.

I don't wake up laughing. I'm coughing my lungs out with the impression my feet have been amputated. *"Oh, my God! They've chopped off my feet instead of fixing my head!"* I struggle to sit up before the mucus chokes me to death. Having conditioned myself to the "horse-snort", I start it automatically and it eases my cough a bit.

Although my feet haven't been amputated, no one can explain why they feel as if they've been skinned. My heels are so sensitive they can barely tolerate a wisp of air touching them. However, after a sympathetic nurse puts a pillow under my legs so my heels don't touch the bed, I feel better. She also adds a few more pillows to support my head and shoulders which helps ease the cough. I feel much better and drift off to sleep only to be awakened again and again by the cough.

I've been left alone in a dark, solitary room lit with just a single light. I'm very cold and very uncomfortable. Strange noises coming from behind pick at my nerves.

"Get a grip!" I tell myself. I fight for control but it's hard not to be scared. *"There, I admit it,*

I'm scared!" It's easy being a smart aleck in a crowd but, alone and confused, I'm scared. I'm utterly terrified of waking up in "The Place" which is only a mile or two north of Loma Linda. I know Dr. Hsu gave me his word but, Jaki and Sue, who have so gallantly given me two years of their lives so I may retrieve mine, cannot be expected to go another round. They have their own lives to lead.

The "horse-snort" and violent coughing brings attention and the news that I'm headed for an MRI. I panic. How can I survive that lying flat on my back with all this junk in my lungs?

The technician, having already dealt with two difficult patients on his shift, doesn't seem to care. In fact, he's downright callous. "You don't have a choice," he states flatly. "Your surgery's in a few hours and this has to be done."

"How long will it take?" I manage to ask between coughs.

"Mmm, about two hours."

"What!" I shriek. "I can't lie flat on my back for two hours! I'll choke to death!"

"Just make sure you don't cough or move when the machine's making a noise," he demands harshly as he rolls me into the "trash compactor", as though I have complete control over my cough mechanism.

This MRI machine is far worse than the one at Moreno Valley. It's like comparing an old Model-T to a Rolls Royce. And the fight not to cough during the clanging noise is a cruel trial.

Even lthough I'm freezing, cold sweat pours off me. *"Calm down, calm down! Nothing lasts forever!" "Yeah, well, five minutes of this is more than forever!"* I argue with myself.

Between coughs, snorts, and the banging MRI, I come to the conclusion that this is probably the worst moment in my life - worse than being held at gun-point by two Turkish soldiers on that remote mountain road near the Bulgarian border. Worse even than losing my shoes and having to wade barefoot over unknown creepy crawlers waist-deep in Amazon muck. And, worse than the time my nearly-mother-in-law came to investigate why the backyard oak tree was bouncing around and her son's and my underwear landed on her head...but, no, that last memory was merely embarrassing, not life-threatening.

I get to the point where I can no longer stand being confined in the "trash-compactor" and scream over the crashing machine to be let out. I'm convinced I'll choke if I lie there another second. The surly technician is not pleased but since I've been in the MRI for an hour and a half he thinks it'll be okay. Okay or not, they'll never get me in that thing again - not tonight, anyway.

It's now almost 3:00 AM and I can't remember ever feeling this exhausted. I wake to find I'm being wheeled into a room crowded with patients being readied for surgery. Everyone there looks pretty miserable. Who can blame them? Like me, they've been deprived of food for who knows how long. All these stomachs sticking to backbones are growling louder than the MRI machine. I'm ready to start chewing on my I.V. tubes.

Being a practical woman who puts basic needs first, my impending surgery has shifted to the non-priority level. All I can think of is food. All I want to talk about is food. Over a day without food! I ask the nurse if there will be dinner waiting when I come around. She gives me a strange look then tells me she'll give me something to calm me down.

"I'm calm and I'm not taking anymore drugs," I tell her. "What I need is to know that I'll have food waiting for me...a good soup...chunky black bread...and some..."

"This is a hospital not a restaurant. Take this and you'll feel better."

"Only food will do that!"

We argue until the good-looking anesthesiologist shows up and takes my side. "She's cool," he tells the nurse. "She practices hypnosis and doesn't need happy pills." I'm given a reprieve from the drugs and soon relax into hypnosis.

It's show time!

But where is Dr. Hsu? The anesthesiologist

assures me Dr. Hsu's on his way. I'd be more comfortable if he were here. I feel like a vulnerable actor deserted by her director on opening night. *"Oh, get a grip, Megan!"* I turn my attention again to hypnosis and gaining control of my cough. I have eight to ten hours of surtery to survive. I don't have time or energy for more drama right now.

I have only vague interest in the technicians scurrying around. A woman brandishing hair clippers announces she's going to give me a shave. I'm vaguely curious as to how I'll look bald.

It's becoming harder and harder to keep my eyes open but I must…I must…see…Dr. Hsu…

My eyes droop.

I'll just close them for a second.

When I open them a minute later Dr. Hsu's smiling face is there in front of me. I'm so happy to see he's arrived. "You can go ahead with the operation," I tell him in a strange, slurring voice.

He squeezes my hand gently. "It all worked out very well."

I'm confused.

"We got it ALL and we had it done in just over six hours."

I reach out to find my head covered with an enormous bandage.

"You finished?"

He nods, still smiling.

"You mean I missed the whole show?"

He gives a little laugh, "Yes! That was on Friday. It's now Monday."

I have difficulty absorbing all the information. Apparently, three days have passed. I have survived the surgery. But have I retained my reading and writing abilities, as meager as they were? My heart chills as I mime my need for pen and paper.

"Later", says Dr. Hsu. "Your brain has been through a very, very difficult time and you must rest."

"No! I must write!" Seeing the fire in my eyes, he reluctantly hands over pen and paper.

I've been practicing this moment for weeks, vowing my first written words would be, "Thank you, Dr. Hsu!" But my hand is weak and my mind befuddled.

I fight to keep calm.

I will not give up. Not now!

I will write this very important thank-you note.

My mind swirls.

I can't quite figure out where to write on the paper and I'm fading fast. I must do something before I pass out. A-B-C is the only thing that flashes to mind. It will have to do for now. I can hardly hold the pen.

"Get a grip!"

Ragged "AB C" crawl onto the paper. I try to give Dr. Hsu a grin as I triumphantly whisper "A, B, C", but my energy is spent. Exaltation hovers in my groggy mind as it sinks into oblivion.

I can still speak!

I can still write!

I can even still read!

I haven't lost it all again. Even though I can't get the words out on paper or even speak them right now, I know that if Dr. Hsu looks into my soul, he will see and hear me saying, *"Thank you!"*

Waking Up

When I next wake Dr. Hsu is gone. I'm in a tiny, dark, windowless area. A single reading lamp lights a small desk where a nurse sits writing. It's quiet except for a faint beep of some machine I'm attached to. I remain tethered to an I.V., a breathing tube in my nose, and other medical accoutrements.

Did I really see Dr. Hsu? Is the operation really over? I tentatively reach up to my head and run my fingers lightly over an enormous bandage. There is no pain, in fact it doesn't even feel as if my head is there at all. It's so creepy I snatch my hand away. I'll deal with it later.

First, FOOD! I'm sure my head will feel better after I've had something to eat. *If it's Monday and I haven't eaten since last Thursday…that means… it's umm…ouch!* A swallow makes my throat feel as if someone's shoveled a handful of broken glass down it. Well, I guess I won't be snacking on the nuts and raisins and my favorite "Hobnob" biscuits Sue stashed in my gym bag.

"Have you anything for me to eat?" I croak to the nurse, startling him. He pushes a food table over my bed with a warning, "Be careful when you swallow. You've had tubes down your throat these last few days." A voice cries out for help behind the curtain near his desk and he disappears.

I blink. My eyes must be playing tricks. The plate of food consists of three cups of chocolate pudding. Only my painful throat stops me howling like a stuck pig. Where's the pureed soup I've been dreaming of for days? I start to push away the poor excuse for food then pull it back. I'm too hungry to be fussy, besides as far as I know it could be midnight with no chance of anything but chocolate pudding till dawn.

Deciding to eat the pudding is one thing, opening the cup is another. My fingers are not at all cooperative. I become desperate. I have to get to the pudding. I must have something in my stomach and start drooling at the thought of eating something. Right now anything will do!

The top flies off the cup and pudding lands all over my face. I scoop it up with my fingers as best I can. It slides down my tormented gullet without too much pain. Not that pain would be any deterrent in my current condition.

I have slightly better luck with the second cup and even attempt to use the spoon. However, it, too, offers difficulties. The pudding first anoints the bandage over my left ear then lands on my nostrils, already burdened with a breathing tube.

Not much success can be claimed for my third effort either. I'm amazed at how far three tiny cups of chocolate pudding can spread, not only on me, but the bed and table, too.

I look up and there stand Jaki and Sue. "You're not supposed to come until Tuesday!" I blurt out, embarrassed they've caught me made-up for Halloween a week too late.

"There's nothing wrong with her," Sue says to Jaki. "She's just as contrary as ever. Not even chocolate pudding's safe around her."

"You looked really terrible yesterday," says Jaki, relief flooding her face.

"So terrible, she was afraid to come alone today," Sue adds.

The nurse, returning to take my vitals, is flabbergasted by the fiasco I've managed to create in just a few minutes.

"Excuse our friend," apologizes Jaki. "We love her but we really can't take her anywhere."

It's terrific to laugh and joke with my friends. I'm so glad they didn't wait another day before coming to see me. However, before I have time to tell them how much it means to me I fall asleep.

Jaki and Sue are gone when I wake and I've been moved to the less intensive part of the I.C.U. My bed overlooks a huge window four flights up. I see the trees below shaking off the last drops of rain. Cars whip up spray from the slick asphalt streets. The setting sun tears loose from the clouds and hurls a double rainbow across the mountains. I stare mesmerized, then bust into laughter.

Life is glorious! And I'm still part of it!

"Can you straighten your head?" asks Dr. Hsu, sounding a little worried when he and Dr. Hadden find me sitting in bed with my head lolling on my right shoulder.

"Well...," I answer with some uncertainty squinting at him sideways, "my head feels weird. Every time I think about the surgery, the hole seems to get bigger and bigger. I can't help imagining all the stuffing falling out of my head if I straighten up."

"You have my word nothing's going to fall out," Dr. Hsu promises.

"I feel like the headless ghost in Harry Potter."

"I assure you, you still have your head. Dr. Hadden opened and closed and he's very reliable, with no record of ever losing a patient's head."

I peer sideways at Dr. Hadden, "Promise you didn't lose...?" I never finish. We all start laughing so much I straighten up without noticing and, sure enough, nothing falls out.

Dr. Hsu settles us down and reaches for the big bandage. "I think we can take this off now."

"No! No, no, no...that's my security blanket. I'm not sure I'm ready to see inside...if I can't feel it how do I know..."

"You have to trust me," challenges Dr. Hsu.

A challenge, especially one from Dr. Hsu, cannot be denied. "Promise me I haven't turned into a headless ghost."

"I promise," he says with a smile and gently removes the bandage. "It might be a year before your sense of feeling returns to the left side of your head and there is a possibility the area around your AVM may always remain a little numb. Your brain has been through a tremendous ordeal. In fact, during the surgery we thought there might be a danger of you having another slight aneurysm. So, I've put you on a different anti-seizure medication to calm your brain down."

"For how long? You know I really want to get off that stuff."

"As soon as we're sure your brain has settled down, we'll get you off it."

"Promise?"

"Yes, I promise."

Dr. Hadden moves in to check his handiwork.

"Did you do a good job?" I ask.

"Would you like to have a look?"

"Mmm...yeeessss," I reply, not at all sure that I really want to. It's a big step for me.

He holds up a mirror. I'm astonished... totally astonished! "How did you do it?" I ask, amazed at what I'm seeing. Except for a long, narrow sliver of missing hair, the rest remains intact. "Now how am I going to impress anyone with a skinny little cut stapled together like a toy? And all the hair's still there. Where's the scar and my bald pate?"

"Is this better?" Dr. Hadden asks with a sly grin and moves the mirror around to show the back of my head.

"Oh, yes, that's more impressive even if it does make me look like a monk," I agree, looking at the shaved circle at the back of my head used to drain the surgical area. In my mind, I see a woodcut of a Benedictine monk that has always fascinated me.

"A hat will easily cover it," Dr. Hadden states, obviously thinking this will comfort me.

Ever the rebel, I laugh and declare, "Cover it? Heck no! I regard it a brand of honor. I'll show it off until it grows out."

I reach for their hands. "I joke because I have no idea how to find the words to thank you for freeing me from those demons growing in my brain and for giving me a new life."

They smile their acknowledgement of my gratitude. We're all quiet a moment, then I announce I'm ready to go home.

"Whoa! It's barely four days after brain surgery and you're still in intensive care..."

"Well, it's your fault I'm feeling so good, Dr. Hsu...and between you and me, I can't hold out a day longer with the food or the noise." I roll my eyes toward the next bed, "Have you ever heard anyone snore like that! She's at it day and night."

Dr. Hsu and I work out a compromise. If I get a green light from all the therapists I can leave Thursday. Of course, I don't admit to anyone that my urge to leave centers on concern for my cat. I still have enough marbles in place to know that would keep me here longer.

I pass the therapists' tests with flying colors. Dr. Hsu honors our agreement and signs my dismissal form. It's now Thursday, Jaki's on her way to pick me up, and I'm being wheeled to the lobby. On the way down I bump into Dr. Siemental. She looks at my head and appears disappointed. "Ohhh…so, you did decide on surgery," she says. I had the very strong feeling I'd let her down, that she had been hoping to provide my treatment. I was beginning to think injured heads were more highly desirable than I'd imagined.

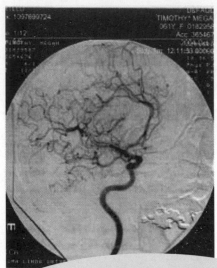

These amazing before (above) and after (below) images of the AVM in Megan's brain show the extent of damage caused by the bleeding artery and the repair done by Dr. Hsu at Loma Linda Hospital.

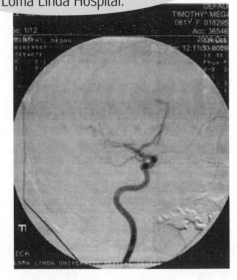

thirty-two

Home Again

Jaki appears tense as she joins me in the lobby. "Don't worry," I tell her, "I'm not going to be a nuisance to you."

"I still don't understand how you talked them into letting you out straight from I.C.U. They always make patients spend at least a couple days in a regular room, you know, just to be sure."

"I zipped through all the therapists' tests and Dr. Hsu declared me 'Wonder Woman'."

"Yeah, great, but does Dr. Hsu know that you live alone?"

"Yes...and he gave me a list of instructions - lots of sleep, as much physical exercise as I can manage comfortably, good food...you know, all the usual recuperation rules."

I have to reassure Jaki again when we reach the car and I nearly topple over getting in. "It's the drugs. They say I'll be staggering around like a drunken sailor for a few more days." Jaki doesn't look entirely convinced I'm ready to leave the hospital. Her lips remain pursed tightly and she frowns during most of the drive back to Hemet. I know she has my best interests at heart, but only I know exactly how I feel and whether I'm ready for this next step. And, I am!

Coon Cat has survived being home alone although her nose is seriously out of joint. I start to give her the saline drip she needs, but only manage about ten minutes before I nearly keel over. A couple of hours of sleep revive me and hot, homemade soup and bread make me feel even better.

The next two weeks are divided between sleeping, eating good food, and walking. Strength flows back. After the first few days I no longer have to use a cane to stop myself from falling over. I'm still performing the horse-snort since my cough continues to plague me, although it, too, has begun to fade. I've started on my reading but find that mental effort is far more draining than any physical exercise.

After two weeks at home, Sue takes me for a check-up with Dr. Hsu. He's delighted at my progress but reminds me to "go slow". "I normally urge all my patients to exercise," he says, "but I'm not going to encourage you. I'm afraid you'll hike up a mountain."

"She already walks a mile and a half every morning", says Sue. "We can't stop her."

"Walking a mile or more is no trouble at all, Doctor, but reading for five minutes knocks me out," I say. "Why would that be?"

"The reading part of your brain was the most damaged and the area I was most concerned about, surgically. It's going to take at least a year or more to recover from the surgery. I can't emphasize enough that you must pay heed to your body. Your body has been through a very difficult period."

"I understand, but please take me off the medication. It's one of the main reasons I had the operation."

Dr. Hsu agrees I can ease off the new anti-seizure medicine but that I'll have to stay on the Neurontin until I've been checked by a neurologist. "Okay, I'll have my nurse come remove the staples. She'll be in in just a moment. Just relax - your brain's not going to fall out." He smiles at our old joke and leaves the room.

The staples come out easily and quickly and we're out of there in five minutes. And, sure enough, my brain is intact.

When we get home, I head immediately for the shower to wash my filthy hair for the first time in two weeks. In the process I discover the nurse missed three more staples. When I show them to Jaki she laughs, and goes to find a pair of pliers. She and I couldn't stop laughing at the comparison between the sterile instruments and environment of the hospital for the first round of staple removal and this last round in the horse barn.

A couple days later we return to Moreno Valley Hospital to see the neurologist. He comes in reading my chart and doesn't so much as give me a glance. "Ah, you had Radiation Therapy at Loma Linda."

"No, I had brain surgery."

"No, dear, you had Radiation Therapy," he

says, tapping my chart while continuing to read.

"No, Doctor, I had brain surgery."

"No," he argues and holds my chart up to me as if speaking to a child, "see, you had Radiation Therapy."

There's no sense in arguing with this man. I just lift up my hair over the large gash in my scalp. His jaw drops and he begins to stammer trying to get some words out. Finally, he blusters, "But...but...you were sent there for...for radiation therapy!"

I stare at him, puzzled. I thought, *"You sent me to Loma Linda for treatment. Why is this a problem?"*

He frantically searches my paperwork, mumbling, "Where's the authorization for surgery? We didn't authorize this. I don't understand..." A couple interns come in to see what the fuss is about and stare first at my head and then at the chart the doctor's holding. They quickly leave. Apparently word has gotten out that I'm now a renegade patient because moments later Dr. K's nurse rushes into the exam room and stares, open-mouthed at my head. She looks dumbfounded and says, "You went to Loma Linda only for radiation therapy. If you'd wanted surgery, you were supposed to have it done here."

I stare at her thinking, *"If I'd known my head was so valuable, I'd have put it up for auction. God knows, I need the money!"*

On the way back to the car, Sue and I stop

and look at each other, reading each other's minds. We realized what a divine intervention had occurred to send me to Loma Linda and Dr. Hsu. What was clearly a human error at Moreno Valley resulted in me getting much better treatment that the Universe apparently meant me to have.

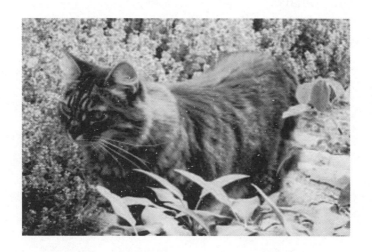

Coon Cat, in her prime.

Goodby Dear Friend

March 15th, 2005

My dear, little Coon Cat died today.

When I return from speech therapy I find she's taken a dramatic turn for the worse and is so weak she can't even turn over. I hold her and stroke her and barely feel her faint purr, but the sound of it has already gone. And a few hours later the rest of her drifts away, too.

A primal, gut-wrenching cry rips through the house and escapes out to the ranch. The sound, so intensely visceral, sets the ranch dogs howling. The unnerving wail holds more tears that are humanly possible, but it's all coming from me. My friend of over twenty years has slipped out of my life.

I suddenly realize that in these last traumatic years it was this frail little creature who has born my grief. I had not allowed myself to mourn my mother's passing, nor to face the reality of my AVM and the terrifying loss of part of my mind and, then, the brain surgery that followed. Piled on top of those traumas came the horror of the fire and stress of my financial crisis. Coon Cat carried these burdens for me. She held the storms at bay. But now that she's gone, I fear the wind will buffet me relentlessly.

All these sorrows bear Coon Cat's name. I can hardly stand to be in my house. She is everywhere and nowhere.

"Oh, my Coonsalayo, my Coonsalayo, where are you?" I moan.

More than a week has gone by and I'm still prone to cry. Soft goodbyes have replaced the wrenching howls but still the pain remains. I have finally said goodbye to my mother. I've relunctantly accepted my brain damage as part of my journey through life. I know I must find the gift hidden within the wretched folds of this experience. Only by doing so will I be able to reclaim my wholeness and sense of well-being. I refuse to remain stagnant in my life but moving forward requires accepting all that has happened up to this very moment.

Slowly my sleep returns to peace and drives away all that has tormented me. Coon Cat rests in the rose garden under the window below my bed, or her bed, as she would have corrected me.

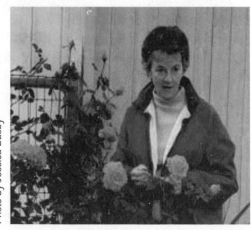

Photo by Jessica Busby

Money!

My four-month penance is over and Sue and I prepare to face the Wicked Witch of Social Security. Sue hopes my recovery from brain surgery will help oil the wheels of Disability Insurance. I suggest she give my "monk" hairstyle a trim since it's begun to lose its eye-caching appearance now that it's started to grow back. Sue gives me a look and tells me she's not shaving my head and if I show up in slept-in clothes again, looking like a homeless person, I'm not riding in her car.

Homelessness is no longer a joke for me. It's almost reality. A month and a half from now the rent money put aside will have evaporated. All I have left is a bicycle and a few clothes.

I'm relieved Coon Cat is gone. She wasn't the kind of cat who'd take kindly to riding around on a bike and living in a tent. I drive these edgy thoughts from my mind and concentrate instead on the Wicked Witch who primes herself for battle.

"Your total monthly income is one hundred, thirty-three dollars and seventeen cents?"

"Yes," I answer. She looks at me through squinted eyes.

"Who pays your rent?"

"Her rent," Sue responds, taking over my part of the interrogation, "was paid in advance and is good only for another a month and a half. After that..." Sue just shrugs.

"Where's her family?"

"She has none."

This woman has no interest in the details of my crises as told to her on two previous occasions. She plows ahead. "And, who has been paying her utilities?"

"Megan is very frugal. Her utilities come to about ten dollars a month."

"Impossible!" snorts the Witch.

Sue rummages around in her files and passes the Witch the year's utility statements, adding icily, "She hasn't had the benefit of air conditioning or heat for the past year."

I'm glad I didn't go to the trouble of shaving my head to impress her. This woman is frozen solid and nothing is going to melt a drop from her.

"Telephone," she snaps.

Sue slides the statements to her as she says, "Average, seventeen dollars a month."

"T.V.? What kind of T.V. does she have?"

"No T.V."

"Car?"

"No car."

The frozen Witch is quiet for a while as she searches hopefully for weapons of mass destruction that don't exist. Sue and I stiffen when we see her relax into her unpleasant smile. "There was a fire in your house about a year ago. How did you replace clothes and household items?"

"Friends went through their closets to..."

"How much?"

"Excuse me?" Sue and I both chorus.

"How much are the clothes and household items worth? Any gifts given are counted as income. You can't expect to be supported by friends and the government."

The humiliation is intolerable - absolutely intolerable! Sue, always cool under pressure, is having a tough time. The Witch scribbles something in her notes then continues. "And what about food? Someone must be helping her out. She couldn't be independent on what she gets." Sue and I stare at her speechless. "She can't expect government assistance if her friends are feeding her." Having delivered this ultimatum, she crosses her arms across her ample chest and leans back.

Sue's eyes run across the two hundred plus pounds of Witch crammed into her desk chair and says, "Well...as is obvious by Megan's size, if she has accepted gifts of food they can't have amounted to much."

I wonder how much I would be penalized if the Witch knew that fifty-percent of my food this past year has come through the kindness of Linda, whose family owns the market garden next door where they grow bok choy. I've eaten a lot of bok choy since my AVM. Bok choy soup, bok choy salad, bok choy stir fry, bok choy sandwiches, and a dozen bok choy creations I have yet to name.

The Wicked Witch tries again. "Why doesn't she work?"

Sue's iciness out-does the Witch's by miles. "Megan has suffered serious brain injury through no fault of her own, and only four months ago underwent traumatic brain surgery. She can hardly be expected to hold down a job after all she's just been through. And her ability to..."

This has about as much effect on the old bat as if she'd been told I'd had a hang-nail removed. "We'll have our own medical staff decide how 'severe' it was, or is," she snips.

And, so, we're dismissed.

Sue is fuming when we get to the car. She looks funny when she's mad. Not having much experience at it, her face is confused as to what is expected of it. I start laughing.

"How can you laugh after that? In a month and a half you'll be out of rent without a penny to your name and still recuperating!"

"You mean I'm not going to be handed one of those infamous Welfare Cadillacs and a beach house?"

Hovering between annoyance and laughter, she finally laughs before chiding me, "This is serious, you know."

"I know, but there's still a month and a half before the guillotine drops." I feel a sickening knot in my stomach that I can't quite ignore and can't decide if my laughter is hysteria or just the ridiculousness of my situation.

I feel encouraged. I've been summoned for a medical inspection by the state. Hopefully, this means a step toward being granted Disability. I'm to go before an ophthalmologist, a psychologist, and an MD. Why not a neurologist?

The ophthalmologist is quick. He has me stare into various gadgets, look left, right, up, and down and that's it.

The psychiatrist is a surly man with no time for conversation. Making no effort to hide his boredom, he holds up cards for me to read and pictures for me to identify. What should I do? If I read faster than a disabled person is supposed to I won't get my rent. If I read too slowly they might send me back to "The Place". I'm in such a dither I can barely read or identify a thing.

The MD is a lovely, vivacious woman loaded with boundless energy. We get along fine and she accepts my suggestion that we ask Sue in to help answer some questions I'm having problems with. "You're depressed," the MD declares making it more a statement than a question.

"No, I'm not..." Sue steps on my foot and I remember her telling me "no arguments! Just agree with whatever they say."

It irks me but I shut up and Sue covers for me. "She has reason to be depressed," agrees Sue running though the list of disasters I've collected over the past year.

"After going through all that she's definitely depressed," declares the MD in a tone that rejects any argument. "I recommend she ask her doctor for Paxil. MediCal will pay for it without question."

"Wait a min..." Sue just about breaks my toes to stifle me.

"Thank you for the recommendation, Doctor," says Sue.

"Paxil has done wonders for me," chatters the speeding MD careening along like a runaway freight train. "I've been using it for years and it's helped my daughter a great deal, too."

Good Lord! The inmates are running the asylum. The System doesn't want to give me money to help keep a roof over my head or get back on my feet as a normal human being, but it's right there ready to dole out drugs which I neither want nor need.

A few weeks later, I'm summoned back to Social Security. The Witch, reluctant to be the bearer of good news, has transferred me to Mr. Nice Guy. "You've qualified!" he tells me cheerfully, pushing papers across for me to sign.

"Your benefits are eight hundred dollars a month. Of course, we'll be deducting the hundred, thirty-three dollars and seventeen cents you receive."

"Of course," I respond ironically.

"You'll receive your first payment in about a week."

"Thank you."

Two weeks go by. No check. I call every day for a week and listen to Mr. Nice Guy's message tell me how important my call is and that he'll return it at the earliest opportunity. My rent looms large. It's due in two weeks. I spend another week calling Mr. Nice Guy and jamming his phone mail every day.

I win!

He calls to say the check is on its way. My rent gets paid...two days late but it's paid. I have a roof over my head...for the next month anyway.

This appeared in *Chocolatier* magine and was one of several articles in food magazines that showed Megan's culinary creativity.

LA MAIDA HOUSE CHOCOLATE TRUFFLE CAKE

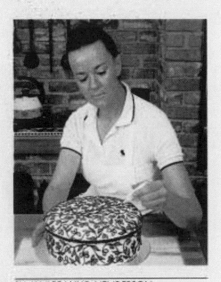

BY JANICE WALD HENDERSON

"What a beautiful piece of porcelain!" exclaims yet another guest at Los Angeles' Spanish-style inn, La Maida House. Stained glass windows, antiques, photographs and paintings abound, but it's a spectacular jewel box that consistently captures the attention of every inn visitor. Resting regally on an antique sideboard, this elegant work of art appears to be made of the finest porcelain. Shimmering like stained glass, an intricate design of intertwining rain-

Janice Wald Henderson writes food and travel articles and teaches food journalism at UCLA.

Megan Timothy, innkeeper and chef at La Maida House in North Hollywood, California, puts the finishing touches on her masterful creation.

thirty-five

Changes

Today I graduate from speech therapy. The thought throws me into a roiling sea of emotion. I'm tossed about by waves of uncertainty and fear. I've grown accustomed to the comfort of working with Alisa. I'm not sure I'm ready to strike out on my own, but the decision is not mine to make. As though I'm a houseguest who has stayed too long, MediCal has let me know I'm no longer welcome in that therapy program.

Alisa assures me I have all the tools I need to continue progressing. She reviews the many battles we've won.

In the beginning I didn't even have a hint of cognitive thought. To all appearances, my brain had stopped functioning. Together with Jaki and Sue we won it back. And we've confronted the "terrible triplets" and won:

Aphasia, the loss of using and understanding spoken and written language -

Agraphia, the cerebral disorder characterized by the inability to write -

And, Alexia, the reader's nemesis.

While we've confronted Alexia, we haven't yet conquered her. Both she and her devilish cousin, Dyslexia, are gremlins who delight in creating the inability to understand written words. Conquering Alexia is my secret to regaining my ability to write. I still can't follow on the computer screen as I'm typing and it's even difficult to track my own handwriting.

Alisa stresses it's imperative that I continue the numbingly repetitive program of sounding out letters and combinations and saying out loud the list of common words I've been adding to every day. Then, there's my new trick of constantly verbalizing everything I see as I go about my daily routines - fence, hose, thyme, sheep, tractor, Colombians, rabbits. All these simple words, still not glued in my brain, require many more hours of repetition to make them stick. However, they are slowly returning to my vocabulary and I'm getting better at calling a strawberry a strawberry and not a tomato.

I'm back to being responsible for myself. While I like the idea of becoming my own person, I'll really miss my sessions with Alisa.

I'm aware my trials are far from over. Alisa warns me that during the first year of recovery from brain damage regaining the basics is relatively fast progression. "After that," she says, "the pace slows down and from now on your progress is going to require even more discipline to reach your goals."

"That doesn't make sense," I argue. "Surely, as I'm regaining knowledge the pace will increase."

"Sorry, that's not the way it works." says Alisa and warns me not to fret or blame myself if progress is slower than I'm used to. "Remember you were very, very lucky to survive your surgery without acquiring any further drawbacks in your capabilities. Promise me you won't lose that indomitable spirit we all love."

"You mean the one Sue calls my pain in the you-know-what?"

She laughs. We hug and, then, she sets me free. But I'm not alone. I have her as a new friend who I know walks with me.

I still need tutoring. While I have gained some ability to correct myself, I also continue to make mistakes that I don't recognize. I'm excited to discover the Adult Literacy Service branch of the Hemet Public Library.

My heart drops when Lori Eastman, the coordinator, tells me the Service has no volunteers with the knowledge needed to assist a brain damaged person but I'm welcome to use their phonics computer program. Seeing my reluctance, Lori encourages me and spends time showing me how to use the program. It works! The audio corrects my mistakes and that's primarily what I need right now.

I'm proud to have found this place on my own and, since it's only eight miles from home, it's an easy ride there and back on my bike. I can only work on the computer for half an hour at a time since mental work still tires me quickly. On the other hand, the physical exertion of the bike ride doesn't bother me at all.

One morning on my way to the center, a car nearly runs me off the road. When I swear at the driver nothing but a jumble of strange sounds come out of my mouth. I know those sounds. I heard them a year and a half ago. I'm terrified!

The vision in my right eye begins to disappear as if someone is pulling a screen over it. *Calm down, Megan! Get a grip! Breathe deep!*

I'm trembling when I reach the center and slide into the privacy of my booth. I close my eyes and fight for control. *The nightmare can't be coming back! Dr. Hsu said he banished all the demons! But, maybe more are still hiding somewhere in my brain.*

I'm so terrified I've lost it all again, that it's a long time before I have the courage to open my eyes. I blink. Amazingly, my vision is clear. Now, can I speak and be understood? The only thing I can think to say out loud is, "Testing, testing, one, two, three," as if checking a microphone. It works! My words come out loud and clear.

I leave the center early that morning. As soon as I'm out the door the screen slides back down my eye. I test the "microphone" again. It's still okay. I ride home unnerved but without further incident.

When I get home, I call Sue. After she and I talk a few minutes she says, "You'd better start documenting these things in case it's something important that Dr. Hsu will need to know."

"Yeah, you're right," I answer, "but maybe I'm just having my post crisis hysterics now."

"Maybe, but still, Megan, write this stuff down so you can talk with Dr. Hsu about it if it keeps happening. He'll want to know what else was going on and when it happened - you know the kinds of things doctors always ask."

About a month later I'm outside calling the cats and hear those garbled sounds coming out of my mouth again. I go back inside and lie down, fighting to control my panic. When my speech returns to normal twenty minutes later I call Dr. Hsu. He reminds me it's not quite six months since my surgery and that my brain is still healing and adjusting.

"Adjusting?"

"Yes," he responds, "the incidents you've experienced are not unusual; however, if they start happening more frequently, come in and see me."

I'm mollified, but not particularly reassured. I thought I finally had a solid bridge to wholeness under me only to find I'm still on a flimsy suspension bridge over a deep chasm. I realize that Dr. Hsu's assurance comes from his vast experience in treating a myriad of patients with conditions like mine, but my fear is personal and pervasive. I need something concrete to base my hopes for my own future upon.

I need to write!

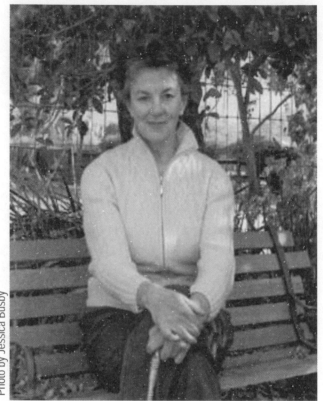

Photo by Jessica Busby

thirty-six

A Book

"Move over, Alexia! There's no room for you in my head!" It's time for real writing. Time to unravel the story of my AVM lying strewn around my mind like the beads of a broken necklace.

It's a mess! How am I ever going to put it together on paper?

Alexia laughs spitefully.

I start to sort out the chaos letter by letter, printing carefully one word at a time in the notebook Sue gave me. Progress screeches to a halt when I try to weave words into sentences. My slow Alexia reading speed can't keep up with my swifter thoughts and writing speed. It's like driving eighty on a freeway trying to dodge all the old farts driving forty-five. Oh, Alexia's having fun with me!

My frustration grows as I rip up page after page. It's as if all the information stored in my head has been run through a paper shredder. *"Calm down, Megan! Think! Make a plan!"*

Yes, I need a plan. I can write down ideas that come out of my mind but it is the reading and editing of them that is almost impossible. *"Work it out! Slowly now!"* No one said it would be easy. I take a deep breath and think.

I learned to read <u>Harry Potter</u> by using the audio tape to guide me. Why not use my memory as I did the audio tape? Laborious as it is, I start by memorizing a single sentence stored in my mind. Then I play around with the words until the construction and sound of the sentence please me. Only then do I write it down, then proceed to the next one. As crazy as it seems, it works. Loosing my sanity is tempting except that I can't afford it. Right now, this is the only way I know to achieve my goal.

Just when I think I have a system for writing worked out, Alexia sneaks in a major blow. She has outlawed my use of the dictionary and thesaurus by making it nearly impossible to comprehend what I'm reading in them. It's like being hit with a two-by-four.

"Get out of my head you witch," I yell.

Alexia just laughs. I almost hyperventilate, I'm so angry.

"Stop being so childish, Megan! Think! Alexia doesn't control your thoughts, you do! Alexia denies the words you most want to use, but you do have the simple words you already reclaimed. Think! Be creative!"

Alexia's furious, but I just laugh and give her the finger. Score one for me!

The battle with Alexia continues. It's a brutal war. She doesn't give up easily and I learn to appreciate the smallest victories. They're growing, however. After a couple of months it becomes possible to use the dictionary and thesaurus on a limited scale. I'm thrilled! *"Yes!"*

Jaki knows about my war with Alexia and

constantly offers help. But writing this book is my Parsifalian journey into the deep, dark forest. And my Holy Grail is the written word – my ability to construct a book of written words. Just as Authur's stalwart knight, Parsifal, had to, I must travel the path alone to come out the other side whole.

Selling this book, having it published is not what's important. Knowing that I've written it, that I met my enemy and conquered both her and my worst fears – that is my triumph!

It's almost Thanksgiving and I've completed the book. That's a big enough gift in itself but the icing on the cake is the fact that it's been bought by a publisher!

While I'm still engaged in the battle with Alexia, the completion and sale of the book is a major victory. I laugh at her and shout, "Got ya!"

This is Megan's mode of transportation for her Bike Ride Around America.

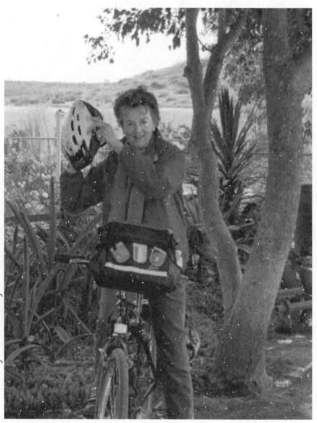

Photo by Jessica Busby

Fun!

I feel pretty cocky after the successful completion of my book. "It's time I had some fun," I announce to Jaki and Sue.

They're pleased to hear it until I confess my idea of fun is a solo bike ride eleven-thousand miles around the country. Sue declares I'm mad, Jaki worriedly suggests I start out with a trial trip maybe to Arizona or north to the wine country.

"You know I've never been one for short trips," I remind them. "Besides this isn't just a casual whim. I have a serious need to prove to myself that I'm whole again."

"Circumventing the country..." moans Jaki.

"Just how do you intend you find your way? Good Lord! How on earth are you going to read maps?" demands Sue.

"I'm sure I'll experience the odd unexpected detour but that's part of the fun of any trip. As long as I remember the sun rises in the east and sets in the west I can't go too wrong."

"But what will you do for money?" Jaki asks, continuing to worry.

"Money...yes...well, now, there is a challenge. I guess it's a good thing I've had so much experience living lean lately."

My friends are somewhat cheered when I promise not to make any hasty decisions until after my up-coming consultation with Dr. Hsu.

Dr. Hsu is happy with the results of my latest angiogram. There's no sign of any monsters lurking in my brain and I haven't had anymore incidents of speech or vision abnormalities. I'm healthy and free to roam.

"Is it okay for me to take a bike ride, then?" I ask, glancing at Sue as I ask the question.

Dr. Hsu smiles, giving me an encouraging nod.

Sue rolls her eyes and says, "She doesn't mean around the block, doctor. She means around the country."

"Where around the country?" he asks her, then looks pointedly at me.

"Eleven-thousand miles around the country!" Sue says pulling out a marked map and holding it up to Dr. Hsu.

Dr. Hsu scans it, his eyes widening. "How many of you...?"

"Oh, no! She's going alone."

"I always go alone. That's the whole point of such an adventure," I tell him.

"But you don't have to go the whole way. You could always..."

"Dr. Hsu, you don't understand," says Sue. "Megan never gives up."

They both look at me. I smile. "No, I never give up." They're not smiling. Dr. Hsu's brow is deeply furrowed. "It's been a year," I say. "My head's pretty well recovered its sensibilities and feels like the head I've always known. I no longer feel like a headless ghost." I grin my famous puckish grin, hoping to put off their concern.

I know a big part of their worry is due to my age, but this fixation on age can really be a millstone. "Look," I say, "I could tell myself, 'My God, Megan, you're sixty-two...old and done for!' And, then I'd feel and behave that way."

"Isn't it better to say, 'Megan, you're sixty-two! Isn't it glorious you have your health, your spirit, and you're off on a grand adventure!'? And then to feel and behave that way?"

Their agreement comes reluctantly. Dr. Hsu continues to frown and Sue mumbles something about me being old and stubborn, but they seem to understand that this decision really is mine, alone, so they can either accept and support me or...

It's a cold, winter night in Southern California. For weeks now I've slept beside an open window attempting to acclimate myself to my upcoming life in a tent. Each night when I wake breathing clouds of fog I come closer to believing Sue and Jaki are right. Maybe I have lost my mind.

Tomorrow I set out on my odyssey. I push the lunacy of it aside replacing it with excitement. Every highway offers unknown destinations, every mountain holds mysteries, and every river sings a different song. And the sky, holding it all together, promises I won't fall off the edge.

I take with me boundless wealth. It lies not in money, but in life, itself. It's not a treasure to horde like gold. My treasure's value increases when it's shared and spread around freely and generously. If you hear me shouting from hilltops on my journey don't be shy. Kick off your shoes and cut loose with me. Don't hold back life - you can't take it with you.

Throw it all into the pot. Stir it up, season it to perfection with laughter, tears, joy, sorrow, heartache, love, hopes, and dreams. Feast on it!

Heck, even life's pits can turn out to taste great!

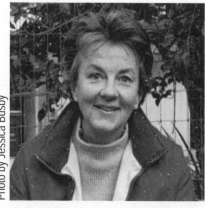

Photo by Jessica Busby

Life is a wondrous feast!

Megan

I WISH TO THANK

NANCY LAYTON, MY PUBLISHER, FOR HER COURAGE IN SUPPORTING AN ALEXIC WRITER WHEN NO ONE ELSE WOULD.

SAMANTHA HORST, LISA FITZGERALD, PAUL WEEKS, AND LORI EASTMAN FOR THEIR PATIENT READING AND GUIDANCE.

MYRIAM GIOVANINNI, ALISA MCFARLAND, DON AND SUZIE NUNLEY, LESLEY ALLEN,

MARGI ALFORD AND LEA PORTER WHOSE ENCOURAGEMENT SUPPORTED ME THROUGH DARK, DARK DAYS.

A FEW GOOD BOOKS

Living With Brain Injury: A Guide for Families and Caregivers; edited by Sonia Griffen Acorn and Penny Offer; published by University of Toronto Press; 1998

Living With Brain Injury: A Guide for Families (2nd Edition); Richard Senelick, M.D. and Karla Dougherty;

I'll Carry The Fork! Recovering A Life After Brain Injury; Kara Swanson; Rising Star Press; 1999 & 2003

Where is the Mango Princess?; Cathy Crimmins; Vintage Books (a division of Random House); 2000

Over My Head: A Doctor's Story of Head Injury From the Inside Looking Out; Andrews McMeel Publishing; 1998 & 2000

AND SOME WEBSITES

Washington:
http://www.headinjury.com

New York:
http://www.bisociety.org

National (with links to affiliate organizations in various states):
http://www.biausa.org

An interesting and informative map of the brain and associated injury related problems:
http://www.neuroskills.com

An informative site by Virginia Commonwealth University (VCU):
http://www.neuro.pmr.vcu.edu

Information specific to vision problems from brain injuries:
http://www.braininjuries.org/

National Organization of Social Security Claimants' Representatives (attorneys who represent people attempting to get Social Security Disability payments) **NOTE**: This site has an EXCELLENT list of questions and answers pertaining to this issue!
http://www.nosscr.org

oma Linda (California) University Medical Center, Neurology Dept. page:
http://www.llu.edu/lluhc/neurosurgery